CONTENTS

Chapter 1: Introduction to Colitis	1
Chapter 2: Anatomy and Physiology of the Digestive System	13
Chapter 3: Types of Colitis	26
Chapter 4: Clinical Manifestations and Diagnosis	66
Chapter 5: Pathogenesis of Colitis	91
Chapter 6: Treatment Approaches	124
Chapter 7: Complications and Prognosis	147
Chapter 8: Preventive Strategies	164
Chapter 9: Future Directions and Research Frontiers	177
Chapter 10: Holistic Health and Colitis Management	185

CHAPTER 1: INTRODUCTION TO COLITIS

Definition and Classification of Colitis

Colitis, derived from the Greek word "kolon" meaning colon and "itis" denoting inflammation, refers to a group of inflammatory disorders affecting the colon and rectum. This condition is characterized by inflammation, ulceration, and often, chronic relapsing nature. Understanding the definition and classification of colitis is pivotal in diagnosing and managing this complex disorder.

Definition: Colitis encompasses a spectrum of inflammatory conditions primarily affecting the large intestine. The hallmark feature is inflammation of the colon mucosa, leading to a range of symptoms including abdominal pain, diarrhea, rectal bleeding, and urgency to defecate. While the exact etiology varies among different types of colitis, the common denominator is an aberrant immune response triggering chronic inflammation.

Classification:

1. **Ulcerative Colitis (UC):** Ulcerative colitis is a chronic inflammatory bowel disease (IBD) characterized by inflammation and ulcers in the innermost lining of the colon

and rectum. It typically involves the rectum and extends proximally in a continuous fashion. The inflammation is superficial, limited to the mucosal layer, and rarely involves the small intestine. UC manifests with symptoms such as bloody diarrhea, abdominal pain, and urgency to defecate. The disease course is marked by periods of exacerbation and remission.

2. Crohn's Disease: Crohn's disease is another form of chronic inflammatory bowel disease that can affect any part of the gastrointestinal tract, from the mouth to the anus. Unlike UC, Crohn's disease involves transmural inflammation, meaning it affects the entire thickness of the bowel wall. This can lead to complications such as strictures, fistulas, and abscesses. Crohn's disease often presents with symptoms similar to UC but can also include extraintestinal manifestations such as joint pain, skin rashes, and ocular inflammation.

3. Microscopic Colitis: Microscopic colitis is a type of colitis characterized by chronic watery diarrhea and normal appearing colon mucosa on colonoscopy. However, microscopic examination reveals inflammation and injury to the colon lining. There are two subtypes of microscopic colitis: collagenous colitis, characterized by a thickened subepithelial collagen band, and lymphocytic colitis, characterized by increased intraepithelial lymphocytes.

4. Ischemic Colitis: Ischemic colitis results from inadequate blood supply to the colon, leading to tissue ischemia and subsequent inflammation. It commonly occurs in the elderly population and is associated with risk factors such as atherosclerosis, hypertension, and hypovolemia. Ischemic colitis typically presents with sudden-onset abdominal pain, bloody diarrhea, and tenderness on physical examination.

5. Infectious Colitis: Infectious colitis is caused by various pathogens, including bacteria, viruses, and parasites. Common causative agents include Escherichia coli, Salmonella, Shigella,

Campylobacter, Clostridium difficile, and Norovirus. Infections can lead to acute inflammation of the colon mucosa, presenting with symptoms such as diarrhea, fever, abdominal cramps, and bloody stools.

6. Radiation Colitis: Radiation colitis develops as a late complication of pelvic radiation therapy for conditions such as pelvic malignancies or gynecological cancers. Radiation damages the endothelial cells and submucosal blood vessels, leading to chronic inflammation and fibrosis of the colon wall. Symptoms include diarrhea, rectal bleeding, and abdominal pain, typically occurring months to years after radiation therapy.

7. Drug-induced Colitis: Certain medications can induce colitis as a side effect. Nonsteroidal anti-inflammatory drugs (NSAIDs), antibiotics, immunosuppressants, and proton pump inhibitors are among the drugs associated with colitis. The mechanism of drug-induced colitis varies depending on the medication but often involves disruption of the gut microbiota, mucosal barrier integrity, or immune modulation.

Conclusion: Understanding the diverse classification of colitis is crucial for accurate diagnosis, appropriate management, and tailored treatment strategies. Each subtype of colitis presents with distinct clinical features, underlying pathophysiology, and therapeutic considerations. A comprehensive approach, considering the patient's clinical presentation, disease severity, and individual factors, is essential for optimizing outcomes in colitis management.

Epidemiology and Prevalence of Colitis: A Comprehensive Overview

Colitis, encompassing various inflammatory conditions of

the colon, poses significant challenges to global healthcare systems due to its chronic nature, potential for complications, and impact on patients' quality of life. Understanding the epidemiology and prevalence of colitis is essential for healthcare planning, resource allocation, and public health interventions aimed at prevention and management.

Epidemiology and Prevalence

Global Burden: Colitis, including ulcerative colitis (UC), Crohn's disease, and other forms, affects millions of individuals worldwide, with varying prevalence rates across different regions. The global burden of colitis has been steadily increasing over the past few decades, likely due to a combination of genetic predisposition, environmental factors, and changes in diagnostic practices.

Regional Variations: Prevalence rates of colitis vary significantly between regions, with higher rates reported in Western industrialized countries compared to developing nations. Regions with a Westernized lifestyle, including North America, Europe, and parts of Asia, have observed a higher incidence and prevalence of colitis. This disparity may be attributed to differences in genetic susceptibility, dietary habits, sanitation, and healthcare infrastructure.

Ulcerative Colitis vs. Crohn's Disease: Ulcerative colitis and Crohn's disease exhibit distinct epidemiological patterns. Ulcerative colitis predominantly affects young adults in their second and third decades of life, with a peak incidence between the ages of 15 and 30 years. In contrast, Crohn's disease often presents in a bimodal distribution, with peaks in incidence during adolescence and early adulthood, as well as in individuals aged 50 to 70 years.

Gender Disparities: Both ulcerative colitis and Crohn's disease demonstrate slight gender disparities in prevalence. Ulcerative colitis has been traditionally associated with a slightly higher prevalence in males, while Crohn's disease shows a slight predilection for females. However, these differences are relatively modest, and the overall prevalence of colitis does not exhibit significant gender bias.

Age-specific Incidence: The incidence of colitis varies with age, with different patterns observed for ulcerative colitis and Crohn's disease. Ulcerative colitis typically presents in younger individuals, with a peak incidence during late adolescence and early adulthood. In contrast, Crohn's disease can affect individuals of any age, including children, adolescents, and older adults, with a second peak observed in individuals aged 50 to 70 years.

Ethnic and Racial Disparities: Ethnic and racial disparities in the prevalence of colitis have been reported, with higher rates observed in certain populations. For example, individuals of Ashkenazi Jewish descent have an increased risk of developing both ulcerative colitis and Crohn's disease compared to the general population. Similarly, African Americans have a higher prevalence of ulcerative colitis compared to Caucasians, while Crohn's disease rates are comparable between these ethnic groups.

Environmental Factors: Environmental factors play a significant role in the epidemiology of colitis, influencing disease incidence and prevalence. Westernized lifestyles characterized by high-fat diets, sedentary habits, smoking, and urbanization have been associated with an increased risk of developing colitis. Additionally, environmental factors such as pollution, industrialization, and hygiene practices may contribute to alterations in the gut microbiota and immune dysregulation, predisposing individuals to colitis.

Temporal Trends: Temporal trends in the prevalence of colitis have shown notable changes over time, reflecting shifts in environmental factors, diagnostic criteria, and healthcare practices. While the incidence of colitis has been increasing in many regions, particularly in newly industrialized countries, there has been a plateau or slight decline observed in some Western countries, possibly due to improved treatment strategies and disease management.

Conclusion: The epidemiology and prevalence of colitis exhibit complex patterns influenced by genetic, environmental, and lifestyle factors. Understanding these epidemiological trends is essential for identifying high-risk populations, implementing preventive measures, and optimizing healthcare delivery for individuals affected by colitis. Continued research into the epidemiology of colitis is crucial for addressing emerging trends and developing targeted interventions to mitigate the global burden of this inflammatory condition.

Etiology and Risk Factors of Colitis: Unraveling the Complex Interplay

Colitis, encompassing various inflammatory disorders of the colon, is a multifactorial condition influenced by a myriad of genetic, environmental, immunological, and microbial factors. Understanding the etiology and risk factors associated with colitis is essential for elucidating disease mechanisms, identifying high-risk individuals, and developing targeted interventions for prevention and management.

Etiology and Risk Factors

Genetic Predisposition: Genetic factors play a significant role in the etiology of colitis, particularly in conditions such as ulcerative colitis (UC) and Crohn's disease. Genome-wide association studies (GWAS) have identified numerous susceptibility loci associated with increased risk of developing colitis. Variants in genes involved in immune regulation, epithelial barrier function, and microbial recognition pathways contribute to disease susceptibility. For example, mutations in the NOD2, ATG16L1, and IL23R genes have been implicated in Crohn's disease, while variants in the HLA region are associated with UC.

Environmental Triggers: Environmental factors play a crucial role in triggering and exacerbating colitis in genetically susceptible individuals. Dietary factors, such as high-fat diets, refined sugars, and low fiber intake, have been implicated in the pathogenesis of colitis. Additionally, environmental pollutants, smoking, stress, and medications such as nonsteroidal anti-inflammatory drugs (NSAIDs) and antibiotics can disrupt the gut microbiota, impair mucosal barrier function, and modulate immune responses, predisposing individuals to colitis.

Dysbiosis of the Gut Microbiota: The gut microbiota, comprising trillions of microorganisms, plays a pivotal role in maintaining intestinal homeostasis and immune regulation. Dysbiosis, characterized by alterations in the composition and function of the gut microbiota, has been implicated in the pathogenesis of colitis. Shifts in microbial diversity, decreased abundance of beneficial commensal bacteria, and overgrowth of pathogenic species can trigger inflammatory responses, disrupt epithelial integrity, and contribute to mucosal inflammation in colitis.

Immune Dysregulation: Colitis is characterized by aberrant immune responses directed against luminal antigens, commensal bacteria, or self-antigens in genetically susceptible individuals. Dysregulation of innate and adaptive immune pathways, including Toll-like receptor (TLR) signaling, Th1/Th2/Th17 cytokine profiles, and regulatory T cell dysfunction, contributes to chronic inflammation and tissue damage in the colon. Immune-mediated mechanisms involving cytokine cascades, chemokine recruitment, and leukocyte infiltration perpetuate mucosal inflammation and drive disease progression in colitis.

Barrier Dysfunction: Intestinal barrier dysfunction, encompassing alterations in epithelial integrity, mucin production, and tight junction proteins, plays a critical role in the pathogenesis of colitis. Disruption of the mucosal barrier allows luminal antigens, microbial products, and toxins to penetrate the intestinal epithelium, triggering inflammatory responses and immune activation. Impaired barrier function predisposes individuals to mucosal injury, bacterial translocation, and chronic inflammation in colitis.

Oxidative Stress and Inflammatory Mediators: Oxidative stress, characterized by an imbalance between reactive oxygen species (ROS) production and antioxidant defenses, contributes to tissue damage and inflammation in colitis. ROS generated by activated immune cells, epithelial cells, and luminal bacteria induce DNA damage, lipid peroxidation, and protein oxidation, exacerbating mucosal injury and inflammatory responses. Inflammatory mediators such as cytokines, chemokines, and eicosanoids further amplify oxidative stress and perpetuate inflammation in colitis.

Lifestyle Factors: Lifestyle factors, including diet, smoking, physical activity, and stress, have been implicated as modifiable risk factors for colitis. High-fat diets, low fiber intake, and consumption of processed foods rich in additives and preservatives are associated with an increased risk of colitis. Conversely, Mediterranean-style diets rich in fruits, vegetables, and omega-3 fatty acids have been shown to exert protective effects against colitis. Smoking has divergent effects on UC and Crohn's disease, with detrimental effects observed in UC and potential protective effects in Crohn's disease. Physical inactivity and chronic stress can exacerbate inflammation and compromise immune function, predisposing individuals to colitis.

Conclusion: Colitis is a complex inflammatory disorder influenced by a multitude of genetic, environmental, immunological, and lifestyle factors. Understanding the etiology and risk factors associated with colitis is essential for elucidating disease mechanisms, identifying high-risk individuals, and implementing targeted interventions for prevention and management. Continued research into the interplay between genetic susceptibility, environmental triggers, and immune dysregulation will provide valuable insights into the pathogenesis of colitis and facilitate the development of personalized therapeutic approaches.

Pathophysiology Overview of Colitis: Insights into Inflammatory Mechanisms

Colitis, encompassing a diverse array of inflammatory conditions affecting the colon, is characterized by a complex interplay of genetic, environmental, immunological, and microbial factors. The pathophysiology of colitis involves dysregulation of immune responses, disruption of mucosal barrier function, alterations in the gut microbiota, and oxidative stress, leading to chronic inflammation and tissue damage. Understanding the underlying pathophysiological mechanisms is crucial for developing targeted therapeutic strategies and improving outcomes in patients with colitis.

Pathophysiology Overview

Immune Dysregulation: The pathogenesis of colitis involves dysregulation of both innate and adaptive immune responses directed against luminal antigens, commensal bacteria, or self-antigens in genetically susceptible individuals. Dysfunctional immune cells, including macrophages, dendritic cells, T cells, and B cells, contribute to chronic inflammation and tissue damage in the colon. Aberrant activation of Toll-like receptors (TLRs), cytokine cascades, and chemokine pathways perpetuates mucosal inflammation and drives disease progression in colitis.

Inflammatory Mediators: Inflammatory mediators, including cytokines, chemokines, and eicosanoids, play a central role in the pathophysiology of colitis. Pro-inflammatory cytokines such as tumor necrosis factor-alpha (TNF-α), interleukin-1 (IL-1), interleukin-6 (IL-6), and interleukin-17 (IL-17) promote leukocyte recruitment, activation of inflammatory pathways, and tissue destruction in the colon. Chemokines such as CCL2, CCL20, and CXCL8 facilitate the migration of immune cells to the site of inflammation, amplifying the inflammatory response in colitis. Eicosanoids, including prostaglandins and leukotrienes, modulate vascular permeability, mucosal blood flow, and leukocyte function, contributing to inflammation and tissue injury in colitis.

Mucosal Barrier Dysfunction: Integrity of the intestinal barrier, comprising epithelial cells, tight junction proteins, mucus layer, and antimicrobial peptides, is crucial for maintaining gut homeostasis and preventing microbial invasion. Disruption of the mucosal barrier allows luminal antigens, microbial products, and toxins to penetrate the intestinal epithelium, triggering inflammatory responses and immune activation in colitis. Impaired barrier function, characterized by alterations in tight junction integrity, mucin production, and antimicrobial peptide expression, predisposes individuals to mucosal injury, bacterial translocation, and chronic inflammation in colitis.

Dysbiosis of the Gut Microbiota: The gut microbiota, comprising a diverse array of microorganisms, plays a critical role in maintaining intestinal homeostasis and immune regulation. Dysbiosis, characterized by alterations in the composition and function of the gut microbiota, has been implicated in the pathophysiology of colitis. Shifts in microbial diversity, decreased abundance of beneficial commensal bacteria, and overgrowth of pathogenic species contribute to inflammatory responses, disrupt epithelial integrity, and promote mucosal inflammation in colitis. Dysbiotic microbiota produce metabolites such as short-chain fatty acids (SCFAs), lipopolysaccharides (LPS), and bile acids, which modulate immune responses, epithelial barrier function, and inflammatory pathways in the colon.

Oxidative Stress and Tissue Damage: Oxidative stress, characterized by an imbalance between reactive oxygen species (ROS) production and antioxidant defenses, contributes to tissue damage and inflammation in colitis. ROS generated by activated immune cells, epithelial cells, and luminal bacteria induce DNA damage, lipid peroxidation, and protein oxidation, exacerbating mucosal injury and inflammatory responses. Inflammatory mediators such as cytokines and chemokines further amplify oxidative stress, perpetuating tissue damage and driving disease progression in colitis.

Neuroimmune Interactions: The gut-brain axis, comprising bidirectional communication between the central nervous system (CNS) and the enteric nervous system (ENS), plays a crucial role in regulating intestinal homeostasis and immune function. Neuroimmune interactions involving neurotransmitters, neuropeptides, and neuroendocrine mediators influence gut motility, secretion, and immune responses in the colon. Dysregulation of the gut-brain axis, characterized by alterations in neurotransmitter levels, neuronal signaling, and stress responses, may contribute to immune dysregulation, barrier dysfunction, and inflammation in colitis.

Conclusion: The pathophysiology of colitis involves a

complex interplay of immune dysregulation, mucosal barrier dysfunction, dysbiosis of the gut microbiota, oxidative stress, and neuroimmune interactions. Elucidating these underlying mechanisms is crucial for developing targeted therapeutic interventions aimed at restoring intestinal homeostasis, modulating immune responses, and attenuating inflammation in colitis. Continued research into the pathophysiology of colitis will provide valuable insights into disease mechanisms and facilitate the development of personalized treatment strategies for patients with this debilitating condition.

CHAPTER 2: ANATOMY AND PHYSIOLOGY OF THE DIGESTIVE SYSTEM

Overview of the Digestive Tract: Understanding the Anatomy and Physiology

The digestive tract, also known as the gastrointestinal (GI) tract or alimentary canal, is a complex system responsible for the ingestion, digestion, absorption, and elimination of food and nutrients. Comprising various organs and structures, the digestive tract functions in a coordinated manner to facilitate the breakdown of food into absorbable molecules and the transport of nutrients to support the body's metabolic processes. An understanding of the anatomy and physiology of the digestive tract is essential for comprehending its role in overall health and the pathophysiology of gastrointestinal disorders.

Overview of the Digestive Tract

Anatomy of the Digestive Tract:

The digestive tract extends from the mouth to the anus and can be divided into several anatomical regions:

1. Mouth (Oral Cavity): The mouth serves as the entry point for food ingestion and initial mechanical and chemical digestion. It contains structures such as the lips, teeth, tongue, and salivary glands, which facilitate chewing (mastication), swallowing (deglutition), and enzymatic breakdown of carbohydrates by salivary amylase.

2. Pharynx and Esophagus: The pharynx is a muscular tube that connects the mouth to the esophagus and serves as a pathway for food and fluids during swallowing. The esophagus is a hollow muscular tube that transports food from the pharynx to the stomach through peristaltic contractions, aided by gravity and the lower esophageal sphincter.

3. Stomach: The stomach is a J-shaped organ located in the upper abdomen, serving as a site for food storage, mechanical digestion, and chemical digestion. It contains gastric glands that secrete hydrochloric acid, pepsinogen, and mucus, facilitating the breakdown of proteins and the conversion of pepsinogen to pepsin for protein digestion.

4. Small Intestine: The small intestine is the longest segment of the digestive tract and consists of three regions: the duodenum, jejunum, and ileum. It is the primary site for nutrient absorption, facilitated by finger-like projections called villi and microvilli, which increase the surface area for absorption. Enzymes from the pancreas and bile from the liver aid in the digestion of carbohydrates, proteins, and fats, while nutrients are absorbed into the bloodstream through the intestinal epithelium.

5. Large Intestine (Colon): The large intestine consists of the cecum, colon, rectum, and anus and is responsible for the absorption of water and electrolytes, as well as the formation and elimination of feces. The colon is divided into segments, including the ascending, transverse, descending, and sigmoid colon, where water absorption and fecal formation occur. Bacterial fermentation of indigestible carbohydrates produces short-chain fatty acids and gases, contributing to colonic motility and fecal bulk.

Physiology of the Digestive Tract:

The digestive process involves several physiological processes coordinated by neural, hormonal, and mechanical factors:

1. **Digestion:** Digestion begins in the mouth with the mechanical breakdown of food by chewing and the chemical breakdown of carbohydrates by salivary amylase. In the stomach, food is further broken down by gastric acid and pepsin, forming chyme. In the small intestine, pancreatic enzymes and bile facilitate the digestion of proteins, fats, and carbohydrates, leading to the release of absorbable nutrients.

2. **Absorption:** Absorption of nutrients occurs primarily in the small intestine, where villi and microvilli increase the surface area for absorption. Nutrients such as glucose, amino acids, fatty acids, vitamins, and minerals are transported across the intestinal epithelium into the bloodstream or lymphatic system for distribution to various tissues and organs.

3. **Motility:** Peristalsis, coordinated muscular contractions, propels food through the digestive tract, facilitating digestion, absorption, and elimination. Segmentation contractions in the small intestine aid in mixing and churning of food, while mass movements in the colon promote fecal transit and elimination.

4. **Secretion:** Gastric glands in the stomach secrete hydrochloric acid, pepsinogen, and mucus, creating an acidic environment for protein digestion and protecting the gastric mucosa. Pancreatic

enzymes, bile acids, and intestinal enzymes are secreted into the small intestine to aid in digestion and absorption of nutrients.

5. Regulation: Neural and hormonal mechanisms regulate digestive processes through feedback loops involving the enteric nervous system, autonomic nervous system, and endocrine system. Hormones such as gastrin, cholecystokinin (CCK), secretin, and ghrelin regulate gastric acid secretion, pancreatic enzyme release, bile secretion, and appetite control.

Conclusion: The digestive tract is a highly specialized system responsible for the breakdown, absorption, and assimilation of nutrients essential for maintaining health and vitality. Understanding the anatomy and physiology of the digestive tract provides insights into its role in metabolism, nutrition, and gastrointestinal function, aiding in the diagnosis and management of digestive disorders and promoting overall well-being. Continued research into the intricate mechanisms governing digestive processes will enhance our understanding of gastrointestinal physiology and inform novel therapeutic approaches for gastrointestinal diseases.

Structure and Function of the Large Intestine:

The large intestine, or colon, is a vital part of the digestive system, responsible for several essential functions in the process of digestion, absorption, and elimination. Understanding its structure and function is crucial in comprehending its role in maintaining overall gastrointestinal health.

Structure of the Large Intestine:

The large intestine is a tube-like organ that extends from the end of the small intestine to the anus. It consists of several anatomical regions, each with distinct structural characteristics:

1. **Cecum:**
   - The cecum is the pouch-like structure that marks the beginning of the large intestine.
   - It receives undigested food from the ileum of the small intestine through the ileocecal valve.
2. **Colon:**
   - The colon is the longest part of the large intestine, divided into four main segments: the ascending colon, transverse colon, descending colon, and sigmoid colon.
   - It functions to absorb water and electrolytes from the undigested food matter, consolidating it into feces for elimination.
   - The colon has a rich blood supply, allowing for efficient absorption of nutrients and water.
3. **Rectum:**
   - The rectum is the final segment of the large intestine, leading to the anus.
   - It serves as a reservoir for feces before defecation, allowing for voluntary control over bowel movements.
4. **Anus:**
   - The anus is the external opening at the end of the digestive tract, through which feces are expelled from the body.
   - It is surrounded by two sphincter muscles, the internal anal sphincter (involuntary) and the external anal sphincter (voluntary), which regulate the passage of feces.

Function of the Large Intestine:

The large intestine performs several important functions in the digestive process, including:

1. **Water and Electrolyte Absorption:**
   - One of the primary functions of the large intestine is to absorb water and electrolytes from the undigested food matter.
   - This absorption process helps in maintaining the body's fluid balance and preventing dehydration.
2. **Fecal Formation:**
   - As water is absorbed from the undigested food material, the remaining contents become more solid and form feces.
   - Fecal formation involves the consolidation of waste material, along with undigested food particles, bile pigments, and bacteria.
3. **Microbial Fermentation:**
   - The large intestine is home to a diverse population of beneficial bacteria known as the gut microbiota.
   - These bacteria play a crucial role in fermenting indigestible carbohydrates and producing short-chain fatty acids (SCFAs), which provide energy for the colonocytes and contribute to overall gut health.
4. **Storage and Elimination:**
   - The rectum serves as a reservoir for feces, allowing for temporary storage until it is expelled from the body during defecation.
   - The anal sphincter muscles control the voluntary passage of feces through the anus, ensuring that bowel movements occur at appropriate times.
5. **Immune Function:**
   - The large intestine contains a significant portion of the body's immune system, with specialized immune cells scattered throughout its mucosal lining.
   - These immune cells help in recognizing and responding to harmful pathogens while

maintaining tolerance to beneficial gut bacteria.

Conclusion:

The large intestine plays a vital role in the digestive process by absorbing water and electrolytes, forming feces, facilitating microbial fermentation, and regulating bowel movements. Understanding its structure and function is essential for maintaining gastrointestinal health and preventing digestive disorders. By maintaining a healthy diet, staying hydrated, and promoting a balanced gut microbiota, individuals can support the optimal function of their large intestine and overall digestive system.

Role of the Colon in Digestion and Absorption:

The colon, a major component of the large intestine, plays a crucial role in the digestive process, particularly in the final stages of digestion and absorption. While the small intestine is primarily responsible for absorbing nutrients, the colon serves important functions in water reabsorption, electrolyte balance, and the fermentation of indigestible carbohydrates. Understanding the specific roles of the colon in digestion and absorption is essential for comprehending its overall contribution to gastrointestinal health.

1. Water and Electrolyte Absorption:

One of the primary functions of the colon is the absorption of water and electrolytes from the undigested material passing through it. As the chyme (partially digested food) enters the colon from the small intestine, it contains a significant amount of water along with undigested food particles, fiber, and waste products. The colon's specialized epithelial cells actively absorb water and electrolytes, allowing for the concentration of waste material and the formation of solid feces.

2. Fecal Formation:

The absorption of water by the colon results in the consolidation of waste material into solid feces. By removing excess water from the chyme, the colon transforms it from a liquid state into a semisolid or solid consistency suitable for elimination. This process of fecal formation is crucial for maintaining normal bowel movements and preventing conditions such as diarrhea or constipation.

3. Fermentation of Indigestible Carbohydrates:

The colon is home to a diverse population of beneficial bacteria known as the gut microbiota. These bacteria play a key role in fermenting indigestible carbohydrates, such as dietary fiber, that escape digestion in the small intestine. Through fermentation, these bacteria break down complex carbohydrates into simpler compounds, including short-chain fatty acids (SCFAs) like acetate, propionate, and butyrate. SCFAs serve as an energy source for the cells lining the colon (colonocytes) and play important roles in maintaining gut health and function.

4. Absorption of SCFAs and Other Metabolites:

In addition to water and electrolytes, the colon also absorbs the short-chain fatty acids (SCFAs) produced during fermentation. SCFAs are readily absorbed by the colonocytes and contribute to various physiological processes, including energy production, regulation of electrolyte balance, and modulation of immune function. Furthermore, the colon absorbs other metabolites produced during fermentation, such as gases (e.g., hydrogen, methane) and microbial metabolites (e.g., vitamins, amino acids), which can influence overall health and well-being.

5. Immune Regulation:

The colon is an important site of immune activity, housing a significant portion of the body's immune cells. Specialized immune cells within the colon's mucosal lining help to maintain immune tolerance to harmless antigens, while also mounting immune responses against harmful pathogens. The gut-associated lymphoid tissue (GALT) present in the colon plays a crucial role in immune surveillance and defense, protecting against infections and maintaining gut homeostasis.

Conclusion:

The colon plays a multifaceted role in the digestive process, contributing to water and electrolyte absorption, fecal formation, fermentation of indigestible carbohydrates, absorption of short-chain fatty acids and other metabolites, and immune regulation. By understanding the specific functions of the colon in digestion and absorption, individuals can appreciate its importance in maintaining gastrointestinal health and overall well-being. A balanced diet rich in fiber, adequate hydration, and support for a healthy gut microbiota can help optimize the function of the colon and promote digestive health.

The Gut Immune System: Safeguarding Gut Health

The gut immune system, also known as gut-associated lymphoid tissue (GALT), is a complex network of specialized cells, tissues, and organs that work together to protect the gastrointestinal tract from pathogens, maintain immune tolerance to harmless antigens, and regulate inflammatory responses. This intricate system plays a crucial role in maintaining gut health and overall immune function. Understanding the structure and function of the gut immune system is essential for comprehending its role in gastrointestinal health and its implications for various diseases and conditions.

1. Anatomy of the Gut Immune System:

The gut immune system is distributed throughout the gastrointestinal tract and comprises several components, including:

1. **Mucosa-Associated Lymphoid Tissue (MALT):** MALT is a specialized immune tissue located in the mucosal lining of the gastrointestinal tract. It includes structures such as Peyer's patches in the small intestine and lymphoid aggregates in the colon, which contain immune cells, including T cells, B cells, and antigen-presenting cells (APCs).
2. **Gut-Associated Lymphoid Tissue (GALT):** GALT refers to the collective immune tissue present in the gut, including MALT, mesenteric lymph nodes, and isolated lymphoid follicles. GALT plays a central role in immune surveillance, antigen sampling, and immune response initiation within the gastrointestinal tract.
3. **Intestinal Epithelial Barrier:** The intestinal epithelium serves as a physical barrier between the gut lumen and underlying immune cells. Specialized epithelial cells, such as goblet cells and Paneth cells, produce mucus and antimicrobial peptides that help maintain barrier integrity and prevent microbial invasion.
4. **Microbiota:** The gut microbiota, comprising trillions of microorganisms, interacts closely with the gut immune system. Beneficial bacteria play a crucial role in immune modulation, tolerance induction, and defense against pathogens, while dysbiosis can disrupt immune homeostasis and contribute to inflammation.

2. Function of the Gut Immune System:

The gut immune system performs several key functions essential for gastrointestinal health and immune function:

1. **Immune Surveillance:** The gut immune system constantly monitors the gut environment for invading pathogens, harmful antigens, and aberrant cells. Immune cells, such as dendritic cells, sample luminal contents and present antigens to T cells in MALT, initiating immune responses when necessary.
2. **Immune Tolerance:** The gut immune system maintains tolerance to harmless antigens, including food antigens and commensal bacteria, to prevent unnecessary immune activation and inflammation. Regulatory T cells (Tregs) play a critical role in inducing and maintaining immune tolerance within the gut.
3. **Inflammatory Responses:** In response to pathogens or tissue damage, the gut immune system can mount inflammatory responses to eliminate threats and promote tissue repair. Innate immune cells, such as macrophages and neutrophils, release pro-inflammatory cytokines and chemokines, recruiting immune cells to the site of infection or injury.
4. **Secretory Immunoglobulin A (sIgA) Production:** sIgA is the predominant immunoglobulin isotype in the gut mucosa and plays a crucial role in mucosal immunity. It acts as a first line of defense against pathogens by neutralizing toxins and preventing microbial adherence to the intestinal epithelium.
5. **Interactions with Gut Microbiota:** The gut immune system interacts closely with the gut microbiota, maintaining a delicate balance between immune tolerance and defense. Beneficial bacteria promote immune modulation and tolerance induction, while pathogenic bacteria can trigger inflammatory responses and disrupt immune homeostasis.

3. Implications for Health and Disease:

The gut immune system plays a central role in the pathogenesis of various gastrointestinal disorders and systemic diseases, including:

1. **Inflammatory Bowel Disease (IBD):** IBD, including Crohn's disease and ulcerative colitis, is characterized by dysregulated immune responses in the gut, leading to chronic inflammation and tissue damage. Dysfunctional interactions between the gut microbiota and the immune system contribute to the pathogenesis of IBD.
2. **Infectious Gastroenteritis:** Acute gastroenteritis caused by pathogens such as bacteria, viruses, and parasites triggers immune responses in the gut, leading to diarrhea, abdominal pain, and inflammation. The gut immune system plays a critical role in eliminating pathogens and resolving infection.
3. **Autoimmune Diseases:** Autoimmune diseases affecting the gut, such as celiac disease and autoimmune enteropathy, involve aberrant immune responses against self-antigens in the gastrointestinal tract. Dysregulated immune activation leads to tissue damage and disruption of gut homeostasis.
4. **Metabolic Disorders:** Emerging evidence suggests that the gut immune system influences metabolic processes and may contribute to the pathogenesis of metabolic disorders such as obesity and type 2 diabetes. Dysbiosis and chronic low-grade inflammation in the gut are implicated in metabolic dysregulation.

Conclusion:

The gut immune system is a dynamic and intricate network of cells, tissues, and organs that plays a crucial role in maintaining gut health and overall immune function. By performing essential functions such as immune surveillance, immune tolerance, inflammatory responses, and interactions with the gut microbiota, the gut immune system protects against pathogens, maintains immune homeostasis, and regulates inflammatory processes within the gastrointestinal tract. Understanding the structure and function of the gut immune system provides insights into its role in health and disease and may inform the development of novel therapeutic strategies for gastrointestinal disorders and immune-related conditions.

CHAPTER 3: TYPES OF COLITIS

Ulcerative Colitis: Understanding a Chronic Inflammatory Bowel Disease

Ulcerative colitis (UC) is a chronic inflammatory bowel disease (IBD) characterized by inflammation and ulceration of the colonic mucosa. It is one of the two main subtypes of IBD, the other being Crohn's disease, and is associated with periods of relapse and remission. UC typically affects the rectum and extends proximally in a continuous fashion along the colon, leading to a range of gastrointestinal symptoms and systemic manifestations. Understanding the pathophysiology, clinical features, diagnosis, and management of UC is essential for providing optimal care to affected individuals.

1. Pathophysiology of Ulcerative Colitis:

The exact cause of UC is not fully understood, but it is believed to involve a complex interplay of genetic, environmental, immunological, and microbial factors. Key features of the pathophysiology of UC include:

1. **Dysregulated Immune Response:** UC is characterized by an inappropriate immune response against luminal antigens or commensal bacteria in genetically

susceptible individuals. Dysregulation of both innate and adaptive immune pathways, including T cell activation, cytokine production, and immune cell recruitment, leads to chronic inflammation and tissue damage in the colon.
2. **Mucosal Inflammation:** In UC, inflammation primarily affects the superficial layers of the colonic mucosa, leading to erythema, edema, and ulceration. Inflammatory infiltrates composed of lymphocytes, plasma cells, and macrophages are present in the lamina propria, along with crypt distortion and crypt abscesses.
3. **Loss of Mucosal Barrier Function:** Disruption of the intestinal epithelial barrier in UC allows luminal antigens, microbial products, and toxins to penetrate the mucosa, triggering immune responses and perpetuating inflammation. Impaired barrier function contributes to mucosal injury and increased susceptibility to microbial invasion.
4. **Altered Gut Microbiota:** Dysbiosis, characterized by alterations in the composition and function of the gut microbiota, has been implicated in the pathogenesis of UC. Shifts in microbial diversity, decreased abundance of beneficial commensal bacteria, and overgrowth of pathogenic species contribute to inflammation and exacerbate disease severity.

2. Clinical Features of Ulcerative Colitis:

The clinical presentation of UC varies widely among individuals and may include:

1. **Bloody Diarrhea:** Bloody diarrhea is a hallmark symptom of UC, resulting from mucosal ulceration and inflammation in the colon. The severity and frequency of diarrhea may fluctuate over time, with periods of remission and exacerbation.
2. **Abdominal Pain and Cramping:** Abdominal pain

and cramping are common symptoms of UC, often occurring during bowel movements or periods of active inflammation. The pain may be localized to the lower abdomen and may be accompanied by bloating or discomfort.
3. **Rectal Bleeding:** Rectal bleeding, manifested as bright red blood in the stool or on toilet tissue, is a characteristic feature of UC. Bleeding may occur intermittently or persistently, depending on the extent and severity of mucosal inflammation.
4. **Urgency and Tenesmus:** Urgency, the sudden and compelling need to defecate, and tenesmus, the sensation of incomplete bowel emptying, are frequently reported symptoms in UC. These symptoms may be exacerbated during periods of active inflammation.
5. **Systemic Symptoms:** In addition to gastrointestinal symptoms, UC can cause systemic manifestations such as fatigue, malaise, weight loss, and fever, particularly during disease flares. These symptoms may reflect the systemic inflammatory response associated with UC.

3. Diagnosis of Ulcerative Colitis:

The diagnosis of UC is based on a combination of clinical evaluation, endoscopic findings, histopathological analysis, and laboratory tests. Diagnostic criteria include:

1. **Clinical Evaluation:** A thorough history and physical examination are essential for assessing symptoms, disease duration, and extraintestinal manifestations. Special attention should be given to gastrointestinal symptoms, family history of IBD, and systemic symptoms.
2. **Endoscopy:** Colonoscopy with biopsy is the gold standard for diagnosing UC. Endoscopic findings typically include mucosal erythema, edema, friability,

ulceration, and loss of vascular pattern. Biopsy specimens reveal characteristic histopathological features of UC, such as crypt distortion, crypt abscesses, and chronic inflammation.
3. **Histopathological Analysis:** Histological examination of biopsy specimens obtained during endoscopy is essential for confirming the diagnosis of UC. Key histopathological features include chronic inflammation, crypt distortion, crypt abscesses, and architectural changes in the colonic mucosa.
4. **Laboratory Tests:** Laboratory tests, including complete blood count (CBC), erythrocyte sedimentation rate (ESR), C-reactive protein (CRP), and stool studies, may help assess disease activity, monitor inflammatory markers, and rule out infectious causes of colitis.

4. Management of Ulcerative Colitis:

The management of UC aims to induce and maintain remission, control symptoms, prevent complications, and improve quality of life. Treatment strategies include:

1. **Medications:** Various medications are used to manage UC, including aminosalicylates, corticosteroids, immunomodulators, biologic agents, and Janus kinase (JAK) inhibitors. These medications target different aspects of the inflammatory cascade and may be used alone or in combination based on disease severity and response to therapy.
2. **Nutritional Therapy:** Dietary modifications, including the adoption of a low-residue diet, avoidance of trigger foods, and supplementation with nutritional formulas, may help alleviate symptoms and support mucosal healing in UC. In severe cases, enteral or parenteral nutrition may be necessary to maintain adequate nutrition.

3. **Lifestyle Modifications:** Lifestyle factors, such as smoking cessation, stress reduction, regular exercise, and adequate hydration, can play a supportive role in managing UC and improving overall well-being.
4. **Surgery:** Surgery may be considered for patients with refractory disease, complications such as toxic megacolon or colonic perforation, or dysplasia or malignancy. Surgical options include colectomy with ileal pouch-anal anastomosis (IPAA) or total proctocolectomy with permanent ileostomy.

Conclusion:

Ulcerative colitis is a chronic inflammatory bowel disease characterized by inflammation and ulceration of the colonic mucosa. The pathophysiology of UC involves dysregulated immune responses, mucosal inflammation, barrier dysfunction, and alterations in the gut microbiota. Clinical features include bloody diarrhea, abdominal pain, rectal bleeding, urgency, and systemic symptoms. Diagnosis relies on a combination of clinical evaluation, endoscopic findings, histopathological analysis, and laboratory tests. Management strategies focus on inducing and maintaining remission, controlling symptoms, and preventing complications through medications, nutritional therapy, lifestyle modifications, and surgery when necessary. By understanding the pathophysiology, clinical features, diagnosis, and management of UC, healthcare providers can provide comprehensive care to individuals with this chronic inflammatory condition and improve their quality of life.

Crohn's Disease: Unraveling the Complexities of a Chronic Inflammatory Bowel Disorder

Crohn's disease is a chronic inflammatory bowel disorder

characterized by inflammation of the gastrointestinal tract. It belongs to the category of inflammatory bowel diseases (IBD), along with ulcerative colitis (UC), but differs in its distribution of inflammation and involvement of deeper layers of the intestinal wall. Crohn's disease can affect any part of the digestive tract, from the mouth to the anus, and is associated with a wide range of symptoms and complications. Understanding the pathophysiology, clinical manifestations, diagnosis, and management of Crohn's disease is essential for providing comprehensive care to affected individuals.

1. Pathophysiology of Crohn's Disease:

The exact cause of Crohn's disease is not fully understood, but it is believed to involve a combination of genetic, environmental, immunological, and microbial factors. Key aspects of the pathophysiology of Crohn's disease include:

1. **Immune Dysregulation:** Crohn's disease is characterized by dysregulated immune responses directed against luminal antigens or commensal bacteria in genetically susceptible individuals. Aberrant activation of both innate and adaptive immune pathways leads to chronic inflammation and tissue damage in the gastrointestinal tract.
2. **Transmural Inflammation:** Unlike UC, which primarily affects the superficial layers of the colonic mucosa, Crohn's disease is characterized by transmural inflammation, involving all layers of the intestinal wall. This can lead to the formation of deep ulcerations, fistulas, strictures, and abscesses.
3. **Granuloma Formation:** Granulomas, aggregates of immune cells including macrophages, epithelioid cells, and multinucleated giant cells, are a characteristic histopathological feature of Crohn's disease. These granulomas can be found in the intestinal mucosa,

submucosa, and serosa, and are indicative of chronic inflammation.
4. **Skip Lesions:** Crohn's disease is characterized by the presence of skip lesions, which are areas of normal or unaffected bowel interspersed with areas of active inflammation. This discontinuous pattern of involvement can make diagnosis and management challenging.

2. Clinical Manifestations of Crohn's Disease:

Crohn's disease can present with a wide range of gastrointestinal and extraintestinal symptoms, which may vary in severity and fluctuate over time. Common clinical manifestations include:

1. **Abdominal Pain:** Abdominal pain, often crampy or colicky in nature, is a hallmark symptom of Crohn's disease. It may be localized to specific areas of the abdomen corresponding to the site of inflammation.
2. **Diarrhea:** Diarrhea is a common symptom of Crohn's disease, resulting from inflammation and disruption of normal bowel function. The stool may be watery, bloody, or contain mucus, and diarrhea may be accompanied by urgency and tenesmus.
3. **Weight Loss:** Chronic inflammation and malabsorption in Crohn's disease can lead to weight loss and malnutrition over time. Decreased appetite, dietary restrictions, and nutrient malabsorption contribute to weight loss in affected individuals.
4. **Extraintestinal Manifestations:** Crohn's disease can affect other organ systems outside of the gastrointestinal tract, leading to a variety of extraintestinal manifestations. These may include joint pain, skin lesions, eye inflammation, oral ulcers, and hepatobiliary complications.
5. **Complications:** Crohn's disease is associated with a

range of complications, including strictures, fistulas, abscesses, intestinal obstruction, perforation, and colorectal cancer. These complications can result from chronic inflammation, tissue damage, and the formation of scar tissue.

3. Diagnosis of Crohn's Disease:

The diagnosis of Crohn's disease is based on a combination of clinical evaluation, imaging studies, endoscopic findings, histopathological analysis, and laboratory tests. Diagnostic criteria include:

1. **Clinical Evaluation:** A thorough history and physical examination are essential for assessing symptoms, disease duration, extraintestinal manifestations, and family history of IBD.
2. **Imaging Studies:** Imaging modalities such as computed tomography (CT), magnetic resonance imaging (MRI), and small bowel series may be used to visualize the gastrointestinal tract, identify areas of inflammation, and evaluate for complications such as strictures or fistulas.
3. **Endoscopy:** Colonoscopy or sigmoidoscopy with biopsy is necessary for visualizing the intestinal mucosa, obtaining tissue samples for histological analysis, and ruling out other causes of gastrointestinal inflammation.
4. **Histopathological Analysis:** Histological examination of biopsy specimens obtained during endoscopy is essential for confirming the diagnosis of Crohn's disease. Key histopathological features include chronic inflammation, granuloma formation, and transmural involvement of the intestinal wall.
5. **Laboratory Tests:** Laboratory tests, including complete blood count (CBC), erythrocyte sedimentation rate (ESR), C-reactive protein (CRP), fecal calprotectin,

and serological markers such as anti-Saccharomyces cerevisiae antibodies (ASCA), may help assess disease activity, monitor inflammatory markers, and differentiate Crohn's disease from other gastrointestinal disorders.

4. Management of Crohn's Disease:

The management of Crohn's disease aims to induce and maintain remission, control symptoms, prevent complications, and improve quality of life. Treatment strategies include:

1. **Medications:** Various medications are used to manage Crohn's disease, including aminosalicylates, corticosteroids, immunomodulators, biologic agents, and Janus kinase (JAK) inhibitors. These medications target different aspects of the inflammatory cascade and may be used alone or in combination based on disease severity and response to therapy.
2. **Nutritional Therapy:** Nutritional support plays a crucial role in managing Crohn's disease, particularly during disease flares or periods of malnutrition. Enteral nutrition, dietary modifications, and supplementation with nutritional formulas may help alleviate symptoms, promote mucosal healing, and support overall health.
3. **Lifestyle Modifications:** Lifestyle factors, such as smoking cessation, stress reduction, regular exercise, and adequate hydration, can play a supportive role in managing Crohn's disease and improving overall well-being.
4. **Surgery:** Surgery may be considered for patients with refractory disease, complications such as strictures, fistulas, or abscesses, or dysplasia or malignancy. Surgical options include bowel resection, strictureplasty, or placement of intestinal strictures, and ileocecal valve removal. Surgery may provide symptom relief and

improve quality of life in select cases of Crohn's disease.

5. **Biologic Therapy:** Biologic agents, such as anti-tumor necrosis factor (TNF) antibodies (e.g., infliximab, adalimumab), anti-integrin agents (e.g., vedolizumab), and interleukin inhibitors (e.g., ustekinumab), have revolutionized the management of Crohn's disease by targeting specific inflammatory pathways. These medications are often reserved for patients with moderate to severe disease or those who do not respond to conventional therapies.
6. **Monitoring and Surveillance:** Regular monitoring and surveillance are essential for assessing disease activity, monitoring for complications, and optimizing treatment strategies in Crohn's disease. This may involve clinical evaluation, laboratory tests, imaging studies, endoscopic evaluation, and histopathological assessment at regular intervals.

5. Complications and Prognosis:

Crohn's disease is associated with a range of complications that can impact prognosis and quality of life. Common complications include:

1. **Intestinal Strictures:** Chronic inflammation and fibrosis in Crohn's disease can lead to the formation of intestinal strictures, causing bowel obstruction and abdominal pain. Strictures may require endoscopic dilation or surgical intervention to alleviate symptoms.
2. **Fistulas:** Fistulas are abnormal connections or tunnels that form between different parts of the gastrointestinal tract or between the intestine and other organs. Fistulas can cause symptoms such as abdominal pain, drainage of pus or stool, and recurrent infections.
3. **Abscesses:** Abscesses are localized collections of pus that can develop within the abdominal cavity or around

the anus in Crohn's disease. Abscesses may cause fever, abdominal pain, and tenderness and require drainage or antibiotic therapy.
4. **Perforation:** Severe inflammation and ulceration in Crohn's disease can lead to bowel perforation, a serious complication associated with abdominal pain, peritonitis, and septic shock. Prompt surgical intervention is required to repair the perforation and prevent further complications.
5. **Colorectal Cancer:** Long-standing inflammation and dysplasia in Crohn's disease increase the risk of colorectal cancer, particularly in patients with extensive colonic involvement or longstanding disease. Regular surveillance colonoscopies with biopsies are recommended to detect dysplasia or early-stage cancer.

6. Conclusion:

Crohn's disease is a chronic inflammatory bowel disorder characterized by inflammation of the gastrointestinal tract. The pathophysiology of Crohn's disease involves immune dysregulation, transmural inflammation, granuloma formation, and the development of complications such as strictures, fistulas, abscesses, and colorectal cancer. Diagnosis relies on a combination of clinical evaluation, imaging studies, endoscopic findings, histopathological analysis, and laboratory tests. Management strategies include medications, nutritional therapy, lifestyle modifications, and surgery when necessary. Regular monitoring and surveillance are essential for assessing disease activity, monitoring for complications, and optimizing treatment strategies. Despite the challenges associated with Crohn's disease, advancements in medical therapy and multidisciplinary care have improved outcomes and quality of life for affected individuals. By understanding the complexities of Crohn's disease and implementing appropriate management strategies, healthcare providers can help individuals with this chronic condition achieve symptom relief, maintain remission, and lead fulfilling lives.

Microscopic Colitis: Exploring a Distinctive Form of Chronic Diarrhea

Microscopic colitis is a type of inflammatory bowel disease characterized by chronic, watery diarrhea and inflammation of the colon, as observed under a microscope. Despite its microscopic nature, microscopic colitis can significantly impact the quality of life of affected individuals due to persistent diarrhea and associated symptoms. Understanding the pathophysiology, clinical features, diagnosis, and management of microscopic colitis is essential for providing appropriate care and improving outcomes for affected individuals.

1. Pathophysiology of Microscopic Colitis:

The exact cause of microscopic colitis is not fully understood, but several factors may contribute to its development:

1. **Immune Dysregulation:** Microscopic colitis is believed to involve dysregulated immune responses in the gastrointestinal tract, leading to chronic inflammation and injury to the colonic mucosa. Immune cells, including lymphocytes and plasma cells, infiltrate the lamina propria and epithelium, contributing to mucosal damage.
2. **Environmental Triggers:** Environmental factors, such as medications, infections, and dietary components, may trigger or exacerbate inflammation in susceptible individuals. Nonsteroidal anti-inflammatory drugs (NSAIDs), proton pump inhibitors (PPIs), and certain antibiotics have been implicated as potential triggers of microscopic colitis.

3. **Altered Intestinal Barrier Function:** Disruption of the intestinal epithelial barrier may allow luminal antigens and toxins to penetrate the mucosa, triggering immune responses and perpetuating inflammation in microscopic colitis. Impaired barrier function may result from genetic predisposition, dysbiosis, or environmental factors.
4. **Dysbiosis:** Alterations in the composition and function of the gut microbiota, known as dysbiosis, have been observed in individuals with microscopic colitis. Changes in microbial diversity, abundance of specific bacterial taxa, and microbial metabolites may influence disease pathogenesis and symptom severity.

2. Clinical Features of Microscopic Colitis:

Microscopic colitis typically presents with chronic, nonbloody diarrhea as the predominant symptom. Additional clinical features may include:

1. **Watery Diarrhea:** Chronic, watery diarrhea is the hallmark symptom of microscopic colitis, occurring multiple times per day and persisting for weeks to months. Diarrhea may be nocturnal or postprandial and may be accompanied by urgency and fecal incontinence.
2. **Abdominal Pain:** Abdominal pain, cramping, and discomfort are common in microscopic colitis, often occurring in association with bowel movements or episodes of diarrhea. The pain may be diffuse or localized to the lower abdomen.
3. **Fatigue:** Chronic diarrhea and fluid loss in microscopic colitis can lead to dehydration, electrolyte imbalances, and fatigue. Fatigue may be exacerbated by disrupted sleep patterns due to nocturnal diarrhea.
4. **Weight Loss:** Severe or prolonged diarrhea in microscopic colitis can result in weight loss and

malnutrition over time. Decreased appetite, nutrient malabsorption, and altered bowel habits contribute to weight loss in affected individuals.
5. **Extraintestinal Manifestations:** Although less common than in other inflammatory bowel diseases, microscopic colitis may be associated with extraintestinal manifestations such as joint pain, skin rashes, and autoimmune conditions.

3. Diagnosis of Microscopic Colitis:

The diagnosis of microscopic colitis is established through a combination of clinical evaluation, endoscopic findings, histopathological analysis, and exclusion of other causes of chronic diarrhea. Diagnostic criteria include:

1. **Clinical Evaluation:** A thorough history and physical examination are essential for assessing symptoms, disease duration, medication use, and potential triggers of diarrhea. Special attention should be given to medications known to be associated with microscopic colitis, such as NSAIDs and PPIs.
2. **Endoscopy:** Colonoscopy with multiple biopsies is the gold standard for diagnosing microscopic colitis. Endoscopic findings may be normal or show nonspecific changes such as erythema, edema, or loss of vascular pattern. Biopsy specimens are obtained from multiple sites throughout the colon and reveal characteristic histopathological features of microscopic colitis.
3. **Histopathological Analysis:** Histological examination of biopsy specimens obtained during colonoscopy is essential for confirming the diagnosis of microscopic colitis. Key histopathological features include chronic inflammatory infiltrates, epithelial injury, and increased intraepithelial lymphocytes or collagen in the lamina propria.

4. **Exclusion of Other Causes:** Other causes of chronic diarrhea, such as infectious colitis, inflammatory bowel disease, celiac disease, and malabsorption syndromes, should be excluded before establishing a diagnosis of microscopic colitis.

4. Management of Microscopic Colitis:

The management of microscopic colitis aims to control symptoms, induce and maintain remission, and improve quality of life. Treatment strategies include:

1. **Medications:** Medications such as budesonide, mesalamine, and corticosteroids may be used to control inflammation and alleviate symptoms in microscopic colitis. Budesonide, in particular, is often considered first-line therapy due to its efficacy and favorable side effect profile.
2. **Probiotics:** Probiotics, such as Lactobacillus and Bifidobacterium species, have been investigated as potential adjunctive therapies for microscopic colitis. These beneficial bacteria may help restore microbial balance and reduce inflammation in the gut.
3. **Dietary Modifications:** Dietary modifications, such as avoiding trigger foods, reducing intake of caffeine and alcohol, and increasing fiber intake, may help alleviate symptoms and improve bowel function in microscopic colitis.
4. **Lifestyle Modifications:** Lifestyle factors, such as stress reduction, regular exercise, adequate hydration, and smoking cessation, can play a supportive role in managing microscopic colitis and improving overall well-being.
5. **Follow-Up and Monitoring:** Regular follow-up and monitoring are essential for assessing treatment response, monitoring for complications, and adjusting

therapy as needed in microscopic colitis. This may involve clinical evaluation, repeat endoscopy with biopsies, and laboratory tests to assess disease activity and treatment efficacy.

5. Conclusion:

Microscopic colitis is a distinct form of inflammatory bowel disease characterized by chronic, nonbloody diarrhea and inflammation of the colon observed under a microscope. The pathophysiology of microscopic colitis involves immune dysregulation, environmental triggers, altered intestinal barrier function, and dysbiosis. Diagnosis relies on a combination of clinical evaluation, endoscopic findings, histopathological analysis, and exclusion of other causes of chronic diarrhea. Management strategies include medications, dietary modifications, lifestyle modifications, and regular follow-up to assess treatment response and monitor disease activity. By understanding the complexities of microscopic colitis and implementing appropriate management strategies, healthcare providers can help individuals with this condition achieve symptom relief, maintain remission, and improve their quality of life.

Ischemic Colitis: Understanding an Acute Bowel Ischemia Syndrome

Ischemic colitis is a condition characterized by insufficient blood supply to the colon, leading to tissue damage and inflammation. It is considered the most common form of acute mesenteric ischemia and can result in a spectrum of clinical manifestations ranging from mild abdominal pain to life-threatening complications such as bowel necrosis and perforation. Understanding the pathophysiology, clinical features, diagnosis, and management of ischemic colitis is crucial for prompt recognition and appropriate intervention to prevent serious complications and improve outcomes for affected individuals.

1. Pathophysiology of Ischemic Colitis:

Ischemic colitis typically occurs due to a reduction in blood flow to the colon, leading to hypoperfusion and subsequent tissue ischemia. Key factors contributing to the pathophysiology of ischemic colitis include:

1. **Vascular Insufficiency:** Ischemic colitis often occurs secondary to vascular insufficiency resulting from acute or chronic reductions in blood flow to the colon. This may be due to arterial occlusion, venous thrombosis, vasospasm, or hypoperfusion related to systemic hypotension or shock.
2. **Atherosclerotic Disease:** Atherosclerosis, a chronic inflammatory condition characterized by the buildup of plaques within arterial walls, is a common underlying cause of ischemic colitis. Atherosclerotic plaques can lead to arterial stenosis or occlusion, impairing blood flow to the colon.
3. **Hypoperfusion:** Conditions that decrease blood flow to the colon, such as hypotension, hypovolemia, heart failure, or vasoconstrictive medications, can predispose individuals to ischemic colitis by reducing perfusion pressure and oxygen delivery to the colon.
4. **Microvascular Dysfunction:** Microvascular dysfunction, including impaired vasoreactivity, endothelial dysfunction, and microthrombosis, may contribute to tissue ischemia and inflammation in ischemic colitis, particularly in the setting of systemic inflammatory conditions or hypercoagulable states.

2. Clinical Features of Ischemic Colitis:

Ischemic colitis can present with a range of clinical features, which may vary in severity depending on the extent and duration of ischemia. Common clinical manifestations include:

1. **Abdominal Pain:** Abdominal pain is the most common symptom of ischemic colitis, typically described as crampy or colicky in nature. The pain may be localized to the left lower quadrant or periumbilical region and may worsen with meals or bowel movements.
2. **Rectal Bleeding:** Rectal bleeding, characterized by the passage of bright red or maroon-colored blood per rectum, is a hallmark feature of ischemic colitis. Bleeding may be intermittent or persistent and may be associated with mucosal ulceration or ischemic injury.
3. **Diarrhea:** Diarrhea is a common symptom of ischemic colitis, typically manifesting as loose or watery stools. Diarrhea may be accompanied by urgency, tenesmus, and fecal incontinence, particularly in severe cases of ischemia or inflammation.
4. **Nausea and Vomiting:** Nausea, vomiting, and anorexia may occur in ischemic colitis, particularly in cases associated with extensive bowel involvement or systemic hypoperfusion. These symptoms may reflect gastrointestinal dysmotility or visceral hypersensitivity.
5. **Systemic Symptoms:** Severe or prolonged ischemic colitis can lead to systemic symptoms such as fever, tachycardia, hypotension, and altered mental status, indicating systemic inflammatory response syndrome (SIRS) or sepsis.

3. Diagnosis of Ischemic Colitis:

The diagnosis of ischemic colitis is based on a combination of clinical evaluation, imaging studies, endoscopic findings, and laboratory tests. Diagnostic criteria include:

1. **Clinical Evaluation:** A thorough history and physical examination are essential for assessing symptoms, risk factors for ischemic colitis, and signs of systemic illness or complications. Special attention should be given to abdominal pain, rectal bleeding, and systemic symptoms suggestive of ischemia or inflammation.
2. **Imaging Studies:** Imaging modalities such as computed tomography (CT) angiography, magnetic resonance angiography (MRA), or mesenteric duplex ultrasonography may be used to assess blood flow to the colon, identify arterial or venous abnormalities, and evaluate for signs of bowel ischemia or infarction.
3. **Endoscopy:** Colonoscopy may be performed to visualize the colonic mucosa, identify areas of ischemia or inflammation, and obtain biopsy specimens for histological analysis. Endoscopic findings in ischemic colitis may include mucosal erythema, edema, hemorrhage, ulceration, or friability.
4. **Histopathological Analysis:** Histological examination of biopsy specimens obtained during colonoscopy is essential for confirming the diagnosis of ischemic colitis and ruling out other causes of colonic inflammation. Key histopathological features include mucosal necrosis, crypt dropout, and inflammatory infiltrates.
5. **Laboratory Tests:** Laboratory tests, including complete blood count (CBC), serum electrolytes, inflammatory markers (e.g., C-reactive protein, erythrocyte sedimentation rate), and coagulation studies, may help assess disease severity, monitor for complications, and guide management decisions.

4. Management of Ischemic Colitis:

The management of ischemic colitis aims to restore blood flow to the colon, alleviate symptoms, prevent complications, and improve outcomes. Treatment strategies include:

1. **Fluid Resuscitation:** Intravenous fluid resuscitation is essential for correcting hypovolemia, maintaining hemodynamic stability, and optimizing tissue perfusion in ischemic colitis. Crystalloid solutions are typically administered initially, with careful monitoring of fluid status and electrolyte balance.
2. **Anticoagulation:** In cases of ischemic colitis secondary to arterial thrombosis or embolism, anticoagulation with heparin or low molecular weight heparin (LMWH) may be initiated to prevent further thrombus propagation and promote recanalization of occluded vessels.
3. **Supportive Care:** Supportive measures such as bowel rest, nasogastric decompression, pain management, and nutritional support may be necessary to alleviate symptoms and support recovery in ischemic colitis. Enteral or parenteral nutrition may be indicated in cases of severe ischemia or prolonged ileus.
4. **Antibiotics:** Antibiotics may be prescribed empirically in cases of suspected infectious colitis or secondary bacterial overgrowth in ischemic colitis. Broad-spectrum antibiotics with activity against enteric pathogens are typically recommended pending culture results.
5. **Surgery:** Surgical intervention may be required in cases of severe ischemic colitis refractory to medical therapy, complications such as bowel necrosis or perforation, or failure of endovascular interventions. Surgical options may include bowel resection, colostomy, or bowel diversion procedures.

Infectious Colitis: Unraveling the Consequences of Gastrointestinal Infections

Infectious colitis, also known as infectious enterocolitis, is a condition characterized by inflammation of the colon and/or small intestine resulting from an infectious agent. It is a common cause of acute diarrhea worldwide and can range in severity from self-limiting gastroenteritis to severe, life-threatening illness. Understanding the pathogens, clinical features, diagnosis, and management of infectious colitis is essential for appropriate management and prevention of complications.

1. Pathogens Associated with Infectious Colitis:

Infectious colitis can be caused by a variety of infectious agents, including bacteria, viruses, parasites, and fungi. Common pathogens implicated in infectious colitis include:

1. **Bacterial Pathogens:** Bacterial pathogens responsible for infectious colitis include enterotoxigenic Escherichia coli (ETEC), Salmonella spp., Shigella spp., Campylobacter jejuni, Clostridioides difficile (C. difficile), and various species of Vibrio, Yersinia, and Aeromonas.
2. **Viral Pathogens:** Viral infections associated with infectious colitis include norovirus, rotavirus, adenovirus, cytomegalovirus (CMV), and enteric viruses such as astrovirus and sapovirus.
3. **Parasitic Pathogens:** Parasitic infections such as Giardia lamblia, Cryptosporidium spp., Entamoeba histolytica, Cyclospora cayetanensis, and Blastocystis hominis can cause infectious colitis, particularly in regions with poor sanitation or contaminated water supplies.

4. **Fungal Pathogens:** Fungal infections such as Candida spp. and Histoplasma spp. may rarely cause infectious colitis, particularly in immunocompromised individuals or those receiving broad-spectrum antibiotics.

2. Clinical Features of Infectious Colitis:

The clinical presentation of infectious colitis can vary depending on the causative pathogen, host factors, and severity of infection. Common clinical features include:

1. **Diarrhea:** Diarrhea is the hallmark symptom of infectious colitis, typically manifesting as loose or watery stools. The frequency and severity of diarrhea may vary, ranging from mild, self-limiting gastroenteritis to severe, profuse diarrhea with dehydration.
2. **Abdominal Pain:** Abdominal pain and cramping are common symptoms of infectious colitis, often localized to the lower abdomen. The pain may be diffuse or colicky and may be exacerbated by bowel movements.
3. **Fever:** Fever is a systemic manifestation of infectious colitis and may occur in response to the underlying infection or the body's inflammatory response. Fever may be low-grade or high-grade depending on the severity of the infection.
4. **Nausea and Vomiting:** Nausea and vomiting may accompany infectious colitis, particularly in cases of more severe or systemic infection. Nausea and vomiting may contribute to dehydration and electrolyte imbalances.
5. **Blood or Mucus in Stool:** Blood or mucus in the stool, known as hematochezia or mucoid diarrhea, may occur in certain types of infectious colitis, particularly those caused by invasive bacteria or parasites. Bloody diarrhea may indicate mucosal inflammation, ulceration, or tissue

invasion.

3. Diagnosis of Infectious Colitis:

The diagnosis of infectious colitis is based on clinical evaluation, stool studies, and, in some cases, endoscopic evaluation. Diagnostic criteria include:

1. **Clinical Evaluation:** A thorough history and physical examination are essential for assessing symptoms, potential exposures, recent travel, and risk factors for infectious colitis. Special attention should be given to diarrhea, abdominal pain, fever, and systemic symptoms.
2. **Stool Studies:** Stool studies, including microscopy, culture, and molecular testing, are used to identify the causative pathogen in infectious colitis. Stool cultures can detect bacterial pathogens, while molecular testing may be used to detect viral or parasitic pathogens.
3. **Endoscopic Evaluation:** Endoscopy with biopsy may be performed in cases of severe or refractory infectious colitis, suspicion of inflammatory bowel disease, or concern for complications such as colonic perforation or toxic megacolon. Endoscopic findings may include mucosal erythema, edema, ulceration, or pseudomembranes.

4. Management of Infectious Colitis:

The management of infectious colitis focuses on supportive care, symptomatic relief, and, in some cases, antimicrobial therapy. Treatment strategies include:

1. **Fluid and Electrolyte Replacement:** Oral rehydration therapy or intravenous fluids may be necessary to correct dehydration and electrolyte imbalances in infectious colitis, particularly in cases of severe diarrhea or vomiting.

2. **Symptomatic Relief:** Symptomatic relief of abdominal pain, nausea, and diarrhea may be achieved with antispasmodic agents, antiemetics, and antidiarrheal medications such as loperamide or bismuth subsalicylate.
3. **Antimicrobial Therapy:** Antimicrobial therapy may be indicated in cases of bacterial or parasitic infectious colitis, particularly in cases of severe or invasive infection, immunocompromised hosts, or outbreaks of foodborne illness. The choice of antimicrobial agent depends on the suspected pathogen and local antibiotic resistance patterns.
4. **Avoidance of Antimotility Agents:** Antimotility agents such as opioids or anticholinergics should be avoided in infectious colitis, as they may prolong the duration of infection or increase the risk of complications such as toxic megacolon. These agents can impair gastrointestinal motility and delay pathogen clearance, potentially worsening symptoms or prolonging shedding of infectious organisms.
5. **Dietary Modifications:** Dietary modifications may help alleviate symptoms and support recovery in infectious colitis. Clear fluids, bland foods, and a low-residue diet may be recommended during periods of active symptoms to minimize irritation of the gastrointestinal tract and promote hydration.
6. **Antiparasitic Therapy:** In cases of parasitic infectious colitis, treatment with antiparasitic medications such as metronidazole, tinidazole, or nitazoxanide may be warranted to eradicate the causative organism and alleviate symptoms. Follow-up stool studies may be necessary to confirm parasite clearance.
7. **Infection Control Measures:** In outbreaks of infectious colitis, infection control measures such as hand hygiene, food safety practices, and sanitation protocols may be

implemented to prevent transmission of the causative pathogen and contain the spread of infection.

5. Complications and Prognosis:

Infectious colitis can be associated with a range of complications, particularly in cases of severe or untreated infection. Common complications include:

1. **Dehydration and Electrolyte Imbalance:** Prolonged diarrhea and vomiting in infectious colitis can lead to dehydration, electrolyte imbalances, and metabolic disturbances. Prompt fluid replacement is essential to prevent complications such as hypovolemic shock or renal dysfunction.
2. **Colonic Perforation:** Severe inflammation or tissue necrosis in infectious colitis may predispose to colonic perforation, a life-threatening complication associated with peritonitis, sepsis, and multiorgan failure. Colonic perforation requires emergent surgical intervention to repair the defect and prevent further complications.
3. **Toxic Megacolon:** Toxic megacolon is a rare but serious complication of infectious colitis characterized by colonic dilatation, inflammation, and systemic toxicity. Prompt recognition and management are essential to prevent bowel perforation and septic shock in patients with toxic megacolon.
4. **Hemolytic Uremic Syndrome (HUS):** Certain bacterial pathogens such as Escherichia coli O157:H7, which produce Shiga toxins, may cause hemolytic uremic syndrome (HUS) in susceptible individuals. HUS is characterized by thrombotic microangiopathy, hemolytic anemia, thrombocytopenia, and acute kidney injury, and may occur as a complication of severe infectious colitis.
5. **Post-Infectious Sequelae:** Some individuals may

experience post-infectious sequelae following resolution of infectious colitis, including post-infectious irritable bowel syndrome (IBS), reactive arthritis, or Guillain-Barré syndrome. These complications may develop weeks to months after the acute infection and require specific management strategies.

The prognosis of infectious colitis varies depending on the underlying pathogen, severity of infection, host factors, and timeliness of treatment. Most cases of infectious colitis are self-limiting and resolve with supportive care and symptomatic treatment. However, severe or complicated cases may require hospitalization, antimicrobial therapy, and intensive care management. With appropriate management and infection control measures, the majority of individuals with infectious colitis can achieve full recovery without long-term sequelae.

Radiation Colitis: Unveiling the Effects of Radiation Therapy on the Colon

Radiation colitis is a condition characterized by inflammation and damage to the colon resulting from exposure to therapeutic radiation. It is a common complication of radiation therapy for pelvic malignancies such as colorectal cancer, gynecological cancers, and prostate cancer. Understanding the pathophysiology, clinical manifestations, diagnosis, and management of radiation colitis is crucial for optimizing treatment outcomes and improving the quality of life for affected individuals.

1. Pathophysiology of Radiation Colitis:

The pathophysiology of radiation colitis involves complex interactions between ionizing radiation, tissue responses, and inflammatory processes in the colon. Key mechanisms contributing to radiation-induced damage include:

1. **Direct Cellular Injury:** Ionizing radiation damages DNA and disrupts cellular function within the colonic mucosa, leading to apoptosis, cell death, and impaired epithelial regeneration. Damage to epithelial cells, endothelial cells, and submucosal structures contributes to mucosal inflammation and ulceration.
2. **Vascular Damage:** Radiation-induced endothelial injury and microvascular dysfunction impair blood flow and tissue perfusion in the colon, leading to ischemia, hypoxia, and tissue hypoperfusion. Microvascular changes may result in mucosal ulceration, submucosal fibrosis, and impaired wound healing.
3. **Inflammatory Response:** Radiation triggers an inflammatory cascade characterized by recruitment of immune cells, release of cytokines and chemokines, and activation of pro-inflammatory pathways. Chronic inflammation perpetuates tissue injury, fibrosis, and remodeling in the colon, contributing to the development of radiation colitis.
4. **Fibrotic Changes:** Prolonged exposure to radiation promotes fibrotic changes in the colon, including collagen deposition, extracellular matrix remodeling, and tissue fibrosis. Fibrosis can lead to luminal strictures, bowel obstruction, and impaired gastrointestinal motility in individuals with radiation colitis.

2. Clinical Manifestations of Radiation Colitis:

Radiation colitis can present with a spectrum of clinical manifestations, which may vary in severity depending on the radiation dose, treatment modality, and individual patient factors. Common clinical features include:

1. **Diarrhea:** Diarrhea is the hallmark symptom of radiation

colitis, typically manifesting as frequent, loose stools with or without blood or mucus. Diarrhea may be acute or chronic, intermittent or persistent, and may worsen with continued radiation therapy or bowel irritants.
2. **Rectal Bleeding:** Rectal bleeding, characterized by the passage of bright red or maroon-colored blood per rectum, is a common manifestation of radiation colitis. Bleeding may be intermittent or persistent and may range from mild to severe, depending on the extent of mucosal injury.
3. **Abdominal Pain:** Abdominal pain, cramping, and discomfort are common symptoms of radiation colitis, often localized to the lower abdomen or perineum. Pain may be exacerbated by bowel movements, rectal distension, or ingestion of certain foods or beverages.
4. **Tenesmus:** Tenesmus, the sensation of incomplete evacuation or persistent urge to defecate, may occur in radiation colitis due to rectal inflammation, mucosal ulceration, or fibrotic changes. Tenesmus may be distressing and interfere with daily activities and quality of life.
5. **Altered Bowel Habits:** Altered bowel habits such as urgency, fecal incontinence, and nocturnal diarrhea are common in radiation colitis, reflecting disturbances in gastrointestinal motility, rectal sensation, and sphincter function. Bowel symptoms may fluctuate over time and may be exacerbated by dietary factors or emotional stress.

3. Diagnosis of Radiation Colitis:

The diagnosis of radiation colitis is established through a combination of clinical evaluation, endoscopic findings, histopathological analysis, and exclusion of other causes of colonic inflammation. Diagnostic criteria include:

1. **Clinical Evaluation:** A thorough history and physical examination are essential for assessing symptoms, prior radiation therapy, underlying malignancies, and risk factors for radiation colitis. Special attention should be given to bowel symptoms, rectal bleeding, and abdominal pain.
2. **Endoscopic Evaluation:** Colonoscopy with biopsy is the gold standard for diagnosing radiation colitis and assessing the extent and severity of mucosal injury. Endoscopic findings may include mucosal erythema, edema, ulceration, friability, telangiectasia, and luminal strictures.
3. **Histopathological Analysis:** Histological examination of biopsy specimens obtained during colonoscopy is essential for confirming the diagnosis of radiation colitis and ruling out other causes of colonic inflammation. Key histopathological features may include mucosal ulceration, submucosal fibrosis, chronic inflammation, and vascular changes consistent with radiation injury.
4. **Imaging Studies:** Radiographic imaging modalities such as computed tomography (CT) or magnetic resonance imaging (MRI) may be used to evaluate for structural abnormalities, complications such as strictures or fistulas, or extraluminal manifestations of radiation colitis.

4. Management of Radiation Colitis:

The management of radiation colitis focuses on symptomatic relief, supportive care, and prevention of complications. Treatment strategies include:

1. **Symptomatic Relief:** Symptomatic relief of diarrhea, rectal bleeding, abdominal pain, and other bowel symptoms in radiation colitis may be achieved with dietary modifications, medications, and

lifestyle interventions. Antidiarrheal agents, analgesics, antispasmodics, and topical therapies may be used to alleviate symptoms and improve quality of life.

2. **Dietary Modifications:** Dietary modifications such as avoiding irritants, increasing fiber intake, and maintaining adequate hydration may help alleviate symptoms and support bowel function in radiation colitis. Individualized dietary counseling by a registered dietitian may be beneficial for optimizing nutritional intake and minimizing gastrointestinal symptoms.

3. **Topical Therapies:** Topical therapies such as rectal corticosteroids, sucralfate enemas, or mesalamine suppositories may be used to deliver targeted treatment to inflamed or ulcerated areas of the rectum and distal colon in radiation colitis. These agents help reduce inflammation, promote mucosal healing, and alleviate symptoms of proctitis.

4. **Systemic Medications:** Systemic medications such as corticosteroids, immunomodulators, or biologic agents may be considered in cases of severe or refractory radiation colitis. These medications modulate the inflammatory response, suppress immune activation, and promote tissue healing in individuals with persistent or progressive symptoms.

5. **Endoscopic Interventions:** Endoscopic interventions such as argon plasma coagulation (APC), electrocautery, or balloon dilation may be used to manage luminal strictures, ulcerated areas, or bleeding lesions in radiation colitis. These interventions help restore luminal patency, control bleeding, and improve symptoms in select cases.

6. **Surgery:** Surgical intervention may be required in cases of severe or refractory radiation colitis, complications such as bowel obstruction, perforation, or fistula formation, or failure of conservative management.

Surgical options may include bowel resection, diversion procedures, or creation of a colostomy or ileostomy to bypass affected segments of the colon.

5. Complications and Prognosis:

Radiation colitis can be associated with a range of complications that impact prognosis and quality of life for affected individuals. Common complications include:

1. **Chronic Symptoms:** Some individuals may experience chronic or persistent symptoms of radiation colitis despite treatment, including diarrhea, rectal bleeding, abdominal pain, and altered bowel habits. Chronic symptoms can significantly impair quality of life and may require long-term management and supportive care.
2. **Rectal Strictures:** Prolonged inflammation and fibrosis in radiation colitis can lead to the formation of rectal strictures, narrowing of the rectal lumen, and impaired passage of stool. Rectal strictures may cause symptoms such as constipation, tenesmus, and difficulty with bowel movements, necessitating endoscopic dilation or surgical intervention to relieve obstruction.
3. **Fistula Formation:** Radiation-induced tissue damage and ulceration may predispose to the formation of fistulas, abnormal connections between the colon and adjacent structures such as the bladder, vagina, or skin. Fistulas can cause symptoms such as fecal or urinary leakage, recurrent infections, and pelvic pain, requiring surgical repair or diversion.
4. **Bowel Obstruction:** Luminal strictures, adhesions, or fibrotic changes in radiation colitis may lead to partial or complete bowel obstruction, impairing gastrointestinal motility and transit. Bowel obstruction can cause symptoms such as abdominal distension, nausea, vomiting, and constipation, necessitating supportive measures, bowel rest, or surgical intervention.

5. **Perforation and Peritonitis:** Severe inflammation, ulceration, or tissue necrosis in radiation colitis may predispose to colonic perforation, a life-threatening complication associated with peritonitis, sepsis, and multiorgan failure. Colonic perforation requires emergent surgical intervention to repair the defect, control sepsis, and prevent further complications.
6. **Radiation Proctitis:** Radiation-induced injury to the rectum and distal colon may lead to the development of radiation proctitis, characterized by mucosal inflammation, ulceration, and bleeding. Radiation proctitis can cause symptoms such as rectal pain, urgency, and fecal incontinence, requiring conservative management or endoscopic interventions to alleviate symptoms and promote healing.
7. **Secondary Malignancies:** Long-term exposure to therapeutic radiation for pelvic malignancies may increase the risk of secondary malignancies in the colon or adjacent organs. Individuals with a history of radiation therapy should undergo regular surveillance and screening for secondary malignancies to facilitate early detection and intervention.

The prognosis of radiation colitis depends on various factors, including the extent and severity of radiation injury, effectiveness of treatment, presence of complications, and individual patient factors such as age, comorbidities, and functional status. With appropriate management strategies, most individuals with radiation colitis can achieve symptomatic relief, heal mucosal injuries, and maintain a satisfactory quality of life. However, some individuals may experience chronic symptoms or complications that require ongoing monitoring and supportive care. Multidisciplinary collaboration between gastroenterologists, oncologists, radiation oncologists, surgeons, and other healthcare providers is essential to optimize the management and outcomes of radiation colitis.

Drug-induced Colitis: Unveiling the Gastrointestinal Effects of Medications

Drug-induced colitis refers to inflammation and injury to the colon caused by the use of certain medications. It encompasses a diverse array of pharmaceutical agents that can disrupt the normal physiology of the gastrointestinal tract, leading to colonic inflammation, mucosal injury, and gastrointestinal symptoms. Understanding the mechanisms, clinical manifestations, diagnosis, and management of drug-induced colitis is essential for identifying potential culprits, optimizing treatment, and preventing complications.

1. Mechanisms of Drug-induced Colitis:

The mechanisms underlying drug-induced colitis vary depending on the specific medication and its pharmacological properties. Common mechanisms include:

1. **Direct Mucosal Injury:** Some medications exert direct toxic effects on the colonic mucosa, leading to epithelial damage, inflammation, and ulceration. Nonsteroidal anti-inflammatory drugs (NSAIDs), chemotherapeutic agents, and certain antibiotics are examples of drugs known to cause direct mucosal injury in the colon.
2. **Altered Intestinal Microbiota:** Certain medications can disrupt the balance of the intestinal microbiota, leading to dysbiosis, overgrowth of pathogenic bacteria, and mucosal inflammation. Antibiotics, proton pump inhibitors (PPIs), and immunosuppressive agents are implicated in altering the gut microbiota and predisposing to drug-induced colitis.

3. **Hypersensitivity Reactions:** Drug-induced colitis may result from hypersensitivity reactions involving the immune system's aberrant response to medications. Hypersensitivity reactions can manifest as eosinophilic infiltration, lymphocytic colitis, or collagenous colitis, characterized by chronic inflammation and histological changes in the colon.
4. **Ischemic Injury:** Certain medications may impair colonic blood flow or predispose to ischemic injury, leading to mucosal ischemia, hypoxia, and tissue damage. Vasoconstrictive agents, sympathomimetics, and medications with vasospastic properties may contribute to ischemic colitis in susceptible individuals.

2. Clinical Manifestations of Drug-induced Colitis:

Drug-induced colitis can present with a spectrum of clinical manifestations, which may vary in severity and onset depending on the offending medication and individual patient factors. Common clinical features include:

1. **Diarrhea:** Diarrhea is the most common symptom of drug-induced colitis, typically manifesting as loose or watery stools with increased frequency and urgency. Diarrhea may be acute or chronic, intermittent or persistent, and may be accompanied by abdominal pain, cramping, or bloating.
2. **Rectal Bleeding:** Rectal bleeding, characterized by the passage of bright red or maroon-colored blood per rectum, may occur in drug-induced colitis, particularly in cases of mucosal ulceration, inflammation, or vascular injury. Rectal bleeding may be intermittent or persistent and may necessitate further evaluation.
3. **Abdominal Pain:** Abdominal pain, cramping, and discomfort are common symptoms of drug-induced colitis, often localized to the lower abdomen or

periumbilical region. Pain may be colicky, dull, or sharp in nature and may be exacerbated by bowel movements or ingestion of certain foods or medications.
4. **Systemic Symptoms:** Systemic symptoms such as fever, malaise, fatigue, and weight loss may occur in severe or systemic drug-induced colitis, indicating systemic inflammation, infection, or complications such as toxic megacolon or sepsis.

3. Diagnosis of Drug-induced Colitis:

The diagnosis of drug-induced colitis is based on a combination of clinical evaluation, medication history, endoscopic findings, histopathological analysis, and exclusion of other causes of colonic inflammation. Diagnostic criteria include:

1. **Clinical Evaluation:** A detailed history of medication use, including prescription medications, over-the-counter drugs, supplements, and recent changes in medication regimens, is essential for identifying potential culprits of drug-induced colitis. Special attention should be given to the onset and duration of gastrointestinal symptoms, relationship to medication use, and presence of associated systemic symptoms or complications.
2. **Medication Review:** A comprehensive review of the patient's medication history is necessary to identify potential culprits of drug-induced colitis. Common medications associated with drug-induced colitis include NSAIDs, antibiotics, PPIs, immunosuppressive agents, chemotherapeutic agents, and biologic therapies.
3. **Endoscopic Evaluation:** Colonoscopy with biopsy is often performed to evaluate the extent and severity of mucosal injury in drug-induced colitis. Endoscopic findings may include mucosal erythema, edema, ulceration, friability, granularity, or vascular changes

consistent with drug-induced injury.
4. **Histopathological Analysis:** Histological examination of biopsy specimens obtained during colonoscopy is essential for confirming the diagnosis of drug-induced colitis and ruling out other causes of colonic inflammation. Key histopathological features may include crypt distortion, inflammatory infiltrates, epithelial injury, or collagen deposition consistent with drug-induced injury.

4. Management of Drug-induced Colitis:

The management of drug-induced colitis focuses on discontinuation of the offending medication, supportive care, symptomatic relief, and prevention of complications. Treatment strategies include:

1. **Discontinuation of Offending Medication:** The first step in managing drug-induced colitis is discontinuation of the offending medication, if possible. Patients should be instructed to stop taking the suspected medication and avoid any related compounds or classes of drugs that may trigger a similar reaction.
2. **Supportive Care:** Supportive measures such as fluid and electrolyte replacement, dietary modifications, and symptomatic relief of gastrointestinal symptoms may be necessary to alleviate symptoms and promote healing in drug-induced colitis. Patients should be encouraged to maintain adequate hydration, avoid irritants, and follow a bland or low-residue diet as tolerated.
3. **Symptomatic Relief:** Symptomatic relief of diarrhea, abdominal pain, rectal bleeding, and other gastrointestinal symptoms may be achieved with medications such as antidiarrheals, analgesics, antispasmodics, and topical therapies. Pharmacological agents may be used to alleviate symptoms while awaiting

resolution of drug-induced colitis.
4. **Endoscopic Interventions:** Endoscopic interventions such as mucosal biopsy, cautery, or dilation may be indicated in cases of severe or refractory drug-induced colitis, complications such as strictures or bleeding, or diagnostic uncertainty. Endoscopic therapy aims to evaluate mucosal injury, obtain tissue samples, and provide targeted treatment to affected areas of the colon.
5. **Follow-up and Monitoring:** Patients with drug-induced colitis should undergo regular follow-up and monitoring to assess symptom resolution, medication tolerance, and disease progression. Follow-up colonoscopy may be indicated to evaluate mucosal healing, confirm resolution of inflammation, and assess for recurrence of drug-induced injury.

5. Prevention of Drug-induced Colitis:

Prevention of drug-induced colitis involves careful selection and monitoring of medications, patient education, and awareness of potential adverse effects. Strategies for preventing drug-induced colitis include:

1. **Medication Review:** Healthcare providers should perform a comprehensive medication review and assess the potential risks and benefits of prescribed medications, particularly those known to cause gastrointestinal side effects or mucosal injury.
2. **Patient Education:** Patients should be educated about the potential gastrointestinal side effects of medications, including symptoms of drug-induced colitis, and instructed to promptly report any new or worsening gastrointestinal symptoms to their healthcare provider. Patient education should emphasize the importance of adhering to prescribed medication regimens, reporting any changes in symptoms or medication tolerance,

and seeking medical attention for concerns related to gastrointestinal health.
3. **Medication Alternatives:** Whenever possible, healthcare providers should consider alternative medications or treatment regimens that have a lower risk of causing drug-induced colitis. Pharmacological alternatives, dosage adjustments, or non-pharmacological interventions may be explored to minimize the risk of adverse drug reactions.
4. **Medication Monitoring:** Regular monitoring of patients receiving medications associated with drug-induced colitis is essential for early detection of adverse effects, symptom management, and optimization of therapeutic outcomes. Healthcare providers should monitor for changes in gastrointestinal symptoms, laboratory parameters, and medication tolerance during treatment.
5. **Risk Stratification:** Healthcare providers should assess individual patient factors, including age, comorbidities, concurrent medications, and history of gastrointestinal disorders, to stratify the risk of drug-induced colitis and tailor treatment strategies accordingly. Patients at higher risk of adverse drug reactions may require closer monitoring, dose adjustments, or alternative therapies to mitigate the risk of colonic injury.
6. **Multidisciplinary Collaboration:** Multidisciplinary collaboration between healthcare providers, including gastroenterologists, pharmacists, oncologists, and other specialists, is essential for optimizing the management and prevention of drug-induced colitis. Collaborative care facilitates comprehensive medication management, patient education, and shared decision-making to minimize the risk of adverse drug reactions and improve patient outcomes.

6. Complications and Prognosis:

Complications of drug-induced colitis vary depending on the severity of mucosal injury, duration of exposure to the offending medication, and effectiveness of treatment. Common complications include:

1. **Persistent Symptoms:** Some individuals may experience persistent or chronic symptoms of drug-induced colitis despite discontinuation of the offending medication, necessitating ongoing management and supportive care to alleviate symptoms and improve quality of life.
2. **Mucosal Injury:** Prolonged exposure to certain medications may lead to extensive mucosal injury, inflammation, and ulceration in the colon, increasing the risk of complications such as strictures, fistulas, or perforation. Severe mucosal injury may require endoscopic evaluation, biopsy, and targeted therapy to promote mucosal healing and prevent complications.
3. **Recurrence:** Recurrence of drug-induced colitis may occur if the offending medication is reintroduced or replaced with a similar agent, leading to reactivation of mucosal inflammation, symptom recurrence, and exacerbation of colonic injury. Healthcare providers should exercise caution when reintroducing medications associated with previous adverse reactions and consider alternative therapies if appropriate.
4. **Secondary Infections:** Prolonged inflammation and mucosal injury in drug-induced colitis may predispose to secondary infections, opportunistic pathogens, or superinfections in the colon, increasing the risk of complications such as infectious colitis, sepsis, or systemic illness. Prompt recognition and management of secondary infections are essential to prevent further morbidity and mortality in affected individuals.

The prognosis of drug-induced colitis depends on various

factors, including the underlying medication, severity of colonic injury, timeliness of intervention, and individual patient factors. With appropriate management strategies, most individuals with drug-induced colitis can achieve resolution of symptoms, mucosal healing, and restoration of colonic function. However, some individuals may experience persistent symptoms or complications that require ongoing monitoring, supportive care, and collaboration with healthcare providers to optimize treatment outcomes and improve quality of life.

CHAPTER 4: CLINICAL MANIFESTATIONS AND DIAGNOSIS

Symptoms of Colitis: Recognizing the Signs of Colonic Inflammation

Colitis, characterized by inflammation of the colon, manifests through a variety of symptoms that can vary in severity and presentation. Recognizing these symptoms is crucial for timely diagnosis, appropriate management, and optimization of patient outcomes. The symptoms of colitis may include gastrointestinal manifestations as well as systemic signs of inflammation, reflecting the underlying pathological processes affecting the colon.

1. Gastrointestinal Symptoms:

1. **Diarrhea:** Diarrhea is one of the hallmark symptoms of colitis, characterized by loose or watery stools that may be frequent and urgent. Inflammation of the colon disrupts normal bowel function, leading to increased transit time and decreased water absorption, resulting in diarrhea.
2. **Rectal Bleeding:** Blood in the stool, known as rectal

bleeding or hematochezia, is common in colitis and often occurs due to mucosal ulceration or inflammation. The blood may be bright red or maroon-colored and may be mixed with stool or seen on toilet tissue.

3. **Abdominal Pain:** Abdominal pain or cramping is a common symptom of colitis, typically localized to the lower abdomen. The pain may vary in intensity and character, ranging from dull aching to sharp and crampy, and may be exacerbated by bowel movements or relieved by defecation.

4. **Tenesmus:** Tenesmus is the sensation of incomplete evacuation or the urge to defecate despite having emptied the bowels. It is often described as a constant feeling of rectal pressure or discomfort and may be associated with mucosal inflammation or irritation.

5. **Bloating and Gas:** Increased gas production and abdominal bloating are common symptoms of colitis, resulting from altered gastrointestinal motility, bacterial fermentation, and impaired gas absorption in the colon. Patients may experience discomfort, distension, and a sensation of fullness in the abdomen.

6. **Mucus in Stool:** The presence of mucus in the stool, known as mucoid diarrhea, is a characteristic feature of colitis and reflects mucosal inflammation and irritation. Mucus may appear as clear or opaque gel-like material and may accompany diarrhea or bowel movements.

2. Systemic Symptoms:

1. **Fatigue:** Systemic inflammation associated with colitis can lead to fatigue, malaise, and reduced energy levels. Patients may experience generalized weakness, lethargy, and difficulty performing daily activities, which can significantly impact quality of life.

2. **Fever:** Fever is a common systemic manifestation

of colitis, particularly in cases of acute or severe inflammation. Elevated body temperature indicates an immune response to the underlying infection or inflammation and may be accompanied by chills, sweats, and systemic symptoms.
3. **Weight Loss:** Unintentional weight loss may occur in colitis, particularly in cases of chronic or severe inflammation affecting nutrient absorption and metabolism. Patients may experience decreased appetite, malabsorption of nutrients, and alterations in body composition leading to weight loss over time.
4. **Joint Pain:** Some patients with colitis may experience joint pain or arthralgia, which may be inflammatory or autoimmune in nature. Joint symptoms may occur concurrently with colonic inflammation or as extraintestinal manifestations of underlying inflammatory bowel disease.
5. **Skin Changes:** Cutaneous manifestations such as erythema nodosum, pyoderma gangrenosum, or mucocutaneous lesions may occur in patients with colitis, particularly in cases of inflammatory bowel disease. Skin changes may reflect systemic inflammation, immune dysregulation, or complications of colonic inflammation.

3. Additional Symptoms:

1. **Nausea and Vomiting:** Nausea and vomiting may occur in colitis, particularly in cases of severe inflammation, obstruction, or gastroduodenal involvement. Nausea may be exacerbated by abdominal pain, bloating, or gastrointestinal dysmotility.
2. **Anemia:** Chronic or recurrent bleeding in colitis can lead to iron deficiency anemia, characterized by fatigue, weakness, pallor, and shortness of breath. Anemia may result from mucosal ulceration, blood loss, or impaired

iron absorption in the inflamed colon.
3. **Dehydration:** Prolonged diarrhea and fluid loss in colitis can lead to dehydration, electrolyte imbalances, and metabolic disturbances. Patients may experience thirst, dry mouth, decreased urine output, and signs of volume depletion requiring fluid replacement therapy.
4. **Changes in Bowel Habits:** Changes in bowel habits such as constipation, alternating diarrhea and constipation, or urgency may occur in colitis, reflecting alterations in gastrointestinal motility, transit time, and rectal sensation. Patients may experience unpredictable fluctuations in bowel habits, which may impact daily activities and bowel control.

Recognizing the diverse array of symptoms associated with colitis is essential for prompt diagnosis, appropriate management, and optimization of patient outcomes. Healthcare providers should perform a comprehensive evaluation, including clinical history, physical examination, diagnostic testing, and endoscopic evaluation, to identify the underlying cause of colonic inflammation and tailor treatment strategies to individual patient needs. Collaboration between gastroenterologists, primary care providers, and other healthcare professionals is essential for delivering comprehensive care and addressing the multifaceted aspects of colitis management.

Physical Examination Findings in Colitis: Identifying Clinical Signs of Colonic Inflammation

During the physical examination of a patient suspected of having colitis, healthcare providers may detect a range of findings indicative of colonic inflammation. These findings, obtained through abdominal and rectal examinations, as well as assessment of systemic signs, provide crucial diagnostic insights and guide further evaluation and management.

1. Abdominal Examination:

1. **Tenderness:** Palpation of the abdomen may reveal tenderness, particularly in the lower quadrants. The tenderness may vary in intensity and distribution, reflecting the extent and severity of colonic inflammation.
2. **Guarding:** In response to palpation, patients with colitis may exhibit guarding, involuntary tensing of the abdominal muscles. Guarding is a protective response to abdominal discomfort and may indicate underlying inflammation.
3. **Rebound Tenderness:** Release of pressure following palpation may elicit rebound tenderness, exacerbating pain. This finding suggests peritoneal irritation and may signify complications such as perforation or peritonitis.
4. **Abdominal Distension:** Abdominal distension, characterized by bloating or enlargement of the abdomen, may be present in cases of severe inflammation or obstruction. It may result from gas accumulation, fluid retention, or colonic dilation.
5. **Masses or Fullness:** Palpation may reveal masses, fullness, or areas of induration, indicating complications such as tumor, abscess, or stricture formation. Detection of such findings prompts further evaluation to assess for underlying pathology.

2. Rectal Examination:

1. **Rectal Tenderness:** Digital rectal examination may elicit tenderness upon palpation of the rectum and surrounding area. Rectal tenderness suggests inflammation or irritation of the rectal mucosa, a

common feature of colitis.
   2. **Rectal Bleeding:** Presence of blood on the examiner's glove or on rectal examination may indicate mucosal ulceration or inflammation. Rectal bleeding is a hallmark feature of colitis and warrants further evaluation.
   3. **Mucosal Changes:** Visual inspection of the rectal mucosa may reveal abnormalities such as erythema, edema, or ulceration. These findings indicate active inflammation and mucosal injury characteristic of colitis.

3. Systemic Signs of Inflammation:

   1. **Fever:** Patients with colitis may present with fever, reflecting systemic inflammation. Fever may be accompanied by chills or sweats and indicates an immune response to colonic inflammation.
   2. **Tachycardia:** Elevated heart rate may be observed in patients with severe colitis, dehydration, or systemic inflammation. Tachycardia is a compensatory response to increased metabolic demand or circulatory compromise.
   3. **Hypotension:** Hypotension, particularly in severe cases, suggests systemic complications such as sepsis or shock. Hypotension requires prompt intervention to stabilize the patient and address underlying pathology.
   4. **Tachypnea:** Increased respiratory rate may occur in response to metabolic acidosis, hypoxemia, or systemic stress. Tachypnea indicates respiratory compromise and warrants further evaluation.

4. Additional Findings:

   1. **Extraintestinal Manifestations:** Patients with colitis may exhibit extraintestinal manifestations such as joint pain, skin changes, or ocular symptoms. These findings may indicate systemic inflammation or complications of

colonic inflammation.

2. **Perianal Examination:** Assessment of the perianal area may reveal findings such as fistulas, abscesses, or skin tags, particularly in cases of Crohn's disease. Perianal involvement suggests complications requiring specialized management.
3. **Nutritional Status:** Evaluation of nutritional status, including weight changes and signs of malnutrition, is important in patients with colitis. Malnutrition may occur due to decreased dietary intake, malabsorption, or increased metabolic demand associated with inflammation.

Recognition of these physical examination findings is essential for accurate diagnosis, assessment of disease severity, and formulation of an appropriate management plan for patients with colitis. A comprehensive approach that integrates clinical findings with diagnostic tests and imaging studies is crucial for optimizing patient care and outcomes.

Laboratory Tests and Biomarkers in Colitis: Evaluating Inflammatory Markers and Disease Activity

Laboratory tests and biomarkers play a pivotal role in diagnosing and managing colitis by providing valuable insights into the underlying inflammatory processes, disease activity, and response to treatment. These tests aid healthcare providers in assessing the severity of colonic inflammation, identifying potential complications, and guiding therapeutic decisions. Here are some commonly used laboratory tests and biomarkers in colitis:

1. Complete Blood Count (CBC):

- **White Blood Cell Count (WBC):** Elevated WBC count indicates the presence of systemic inflammation, which is commonly seen in active colitis.
- **Hemoglobin (Hb) and Hematocrit (Hct):** Decreased Hb and Hct levels may suggest anemia due to chronic bleeding associated with colonic inflammation or ulceration.
- **Platelet Count:** Thrombocytosis, an elevated platelet count, may occur as a reactive response to inflammation in colitis.

2. **Inflammatory Markers:**

- **C-reactive Protein (CRP):** Elevated CRP levels indicate systemic inflammation and are often used as a marker of disease activity in colitis. Monitoring CRP levels helps assess response to treatment and detect disease flares.
- **Erythrocyte Sedimentation Rate (ESR):** Elevated ESR is another marker of systemic inflammation and can be used to assess disease activity and response to therapy in colitis.

3. **Fecal Markers:**

- **Calprotectin:** Fecal calprotectin is a marker of intestinal inflammation and is elevated in patients with active colitis. Measurement of fecal calprotectin levels helps differentiate inflammatory bowel diseases (IBD) from non-inflammatory conditions and assess response to treatment.
- **Lactoferrin:** Elevated fecal lactoferrin levels indicate the presence of neutrophilic inflammation in the colon and are associated with active colitis.

4. **Serological Tests:**

- **Antibody Testing:** Serological tests, including anti-

Saccharomyces cerevisiae antibodies (ASCA) and anti-neutrophil cytoplasmic antibodies (ANCA), may be used to differentiate between Crohn's disease and ulcerative colitis, the two main types of IBD.

5. Stool Studies:

- **Stool Culture:** Stool culture may be performed to rule out infectious causes of colitis, such as bacterial, viral, or parasitic pathogens.
- **Stool Ova and Parasite (O&P) Examination:** O&P examination helps detect the presence of parasites in the stool, which can cause infectious colitis.

6. Biochemical Tests:

- **Electrolyte Levels:** Measurement of electrolyte levels, including sodium, potassium, and chloride, helps assess for dehydration and electrolyte imbalances associated with diarrhea in colitis.
- **Liver Function Tests (LFTs):** LFTs may be performed to assess liver function and detect hepatobiliary complications associated with colitis, such as primary sclerosing cholangitis (PSC) in patients with IBD.

7. Genetic Testing:

- **HLA Typing:** Human leukocyte antigen (HLA) typing may be used to identify genetic predispositions to certain types of colitis, such as HLA-DQ2 and HLA-DQ8 in patients with celiac disease-associated colitis.

8. Tumor Markers:

- **Carcinoembryonic Antigen (CEA):** Elevated CEA levels may indicate the presence of colorectal cancer or its recurrence in patients with colitis, particularly in cases of long-standing inflammation or dysplasia.

9. **Imaging Studies:**

   - **Endoscopy and Biopsy:** Endoscopic evaluation with biopsy remains the gold standard for diagnosing and assessing the severity of colitis. Biopsy specimens are examined histologically for evidence of inflammation, mucosal changes, and dysplasia.
   - **Radiological Imaging:** Imaging modalities such as computed tomography (CT), magnetic resonance imaging (MRI), and ultrasonography may be used to evaluate colonic inflammation, assess for complications, and monitor disease progression in colitis.

10. **Novel Biomarkers:**

    - **Microbial Markers:** Emerging research focuses on microbial markers, including gut microbiota composition and microbial metabolites, as potential biomarkers for colitis and IBD. These markers offer insights into the role of the gut microbiome in disease pathogenesis and may aid in personalized treatment approaches.

Laboratory tests and biomarkers are integral components of the diagnostic workup and management of colitis. Interpretation of these tests, in conjunction with clinical findings and imaging studies, allows healthcare providers to tailor treatment strategies and optimize patient care for individuals with colitis.

Endoscopic and Imaging Studies in Colitis: Advancing Diagnostic and Therapeutic Precision

Endoscopic and imaging studies play a pivotal role in the comprehensive evaluation, diagnosis, and management of colitis, providing valuable insights into the extent and severity of colonic inflammation, mucosal changes, and potential complications. These diagnostic modalities offer precise visualization of the colonic mucosa, enabling healthcare providers to assess disease activity, monitor treatment response, and guide therapeutic interventions. By combining endoscopic and imaging studies with clinical assessment and laboratory findings, healthcare providers can tailor individualized treatment strategies and optimize outcomes for patients with colitis.

1. Endoscopic Evaluation:

Endoscopic examination, including colonoscopy and flexible sigmoidoscopy, remains the cornerstone of diagnostic assessment in colitis, allowing direct visualization of the colonic mucosa and collection of tissue samples for histological evaluation. Endoscopic findings provide crucial information about the distribution, severity, and extent of colonic inflammation, guiding treatment decisions and prognostic assessment. Key aspects of endoscopic evaluation in colitis include:

- **Mucosal Appearance:** Endoscopic examination reveals characteristic mucosal changes associated with colitis, including erythema, edema, friability, granularity, ulceration, and pseudopolyps. The presence and severity of these mucosal abnormalities help classify the type of colitis and assess disease activity.
- **Extent of Involvement:** Endoscopy enables assessment of the extent and distribution of colonic inflammation, distinguishing between proctitis (limited to the rectum), left-sided colitis (involving the rectosigmoid and descending colon), and pancolitis (affecting the entire colon). This information guides treatment decisions and determines the need for additional diagnostic testing or

surgical intervention.
- **Endoscopic Severity Scores:** Various endoscopic scoring systems, such as the Mayo endoscopic subscore and the Ulcerative Colitis Endoscopic Index of Severity (UCEIS), quantify the severity of mucosal inflammation and guide treatment response assessment in ulcerative colitis. Endoscopic remission, defined by normalization of mucosal appearance, is a key treatment target in colitis management.
- **Dysplasia Surveillance:** Patients with long-standing colitis, particularly those with inflammatory bowel disease (IBD), require regular surveillance colonoscopy to detect dysplasia or early neoplastic changes. Endoscopic surveillance protocols, incorporating targeted biopsies, chromoendoscopy, and advanced imaging techniques, aim to detect dysplasia at an early stage and reduce the risk of colorectal cancer.

2. Imaging Studies:

In addition to endoscopy, various imaging modalities are employed to assess colitis, evaluate complications, and guide therapeutic decisions. Radiological imaging complements endoscopic evaluation, providing information about extraluminal changes, disease extent, and associated complications. Key imaging studies in colitis include:

- **Computed Tomography (CT):** Abdominal CT imaging is widely used in the evaluation of colitis, particularly in cases of acute exacerbation, suspected complications, or surgical planning. CT findings may include colonic wall thickening, pericolonic fat stranding, bowel dilation, mesenteric lymphadenopathy, and extraluminal collections suggestive of abscess or perforation.
- **Magnetic Resonance Imaging (MRI):** MRI with contrast enhancement is increasingly utilized for

colitis evaluation, offering excellent soft tissue contrast and multiplanar imaging capabilities without ionizing radiation. MRI findings in colitis may include mural thickening, mucosal enhancement, T2 hyperintensity, and perianal involvement, aiding in disease characterization and treatment planning.

- **Ultrasound (US):** Abdominal ultrasound is a non-invasive imaging modality used to evaluate colonic inflammation, assess for complications such as abscess or fistula, and guide therapeutic interventions such as percutaneous drainage. Ultrasound findings may include bowel wall thickening, hyperemia on Doppler imaging, and adjacent fluid collections indicative of inflammation or abscess.
- **Endoscopic Ultrasound (EUS):** Endoscopic ultrasound combines endoscopic and ultrasound imaging techniques to assess colonic wall layers, pericolonic structures, and regional lymph nodes. EUS facilitates accurate staging of colonic tumors, assessment of mural inflammation, and detection of perirectal or perianal complications in colitis.
- **Capsule Endoscopy:** Wireless capsule endoscopy allows visualization of the entire small intestine and selected segments of the colon, providing valuable diagnostic information in patients with suspected small bowel or colonic involvement. Capsule endoscopy may be used in cases of unexplained gastrointestinal bleeding, suspected Crohn's disease, or evaluation of colonic inflammation.

3. Advanced Endoscopic Techniques:

In addition to conventional endoscopy, advanced endoscopic techniques offer enhanced visualization, tissue sampling, and therapeutic interventions in colitis. These techniques, including chromoendoscopy, narrow-band imaging (NBI), confocal laser endomicroscopy (CLE), and endoscopic mucosal resection

(EMR), enhance diagnostic accuracy, enable targeted biopsies, and facilitate minimally invasive treatment of colonic lesions. Key applications of advanced endoscopic techniques in colitis include:

- **Chromoendoscopy:** Chromoendoscopy involves topical application of contrast agents, such as indigo carmine or methylene blue, to enhance mucosal visualization and delineate subtle changes in colonic architecture. Chromoendoscopy improves detection of dysplasia, guides targeted biopsies, and aids in surveillance of colitis-associated neoplasia.
- **Narrow-Band Imaging (NBI):** NBI utilizes narrow-band light filters to enhance visualization of mucosal vascular patterns, facilitating detection of subtle mucosal abnormalities and prediction of disease severity in colitis. NBI improves lesion characterization, reduces the need for random biopsies, and enhances diagnostic yield in colonic evaluation.
- **Confocal Laser Endomicroscopy (CLE):** CLE enables real-time microscopic imaging of the colonic mucosa at cellular resolution, allowing direct visualization of inflammatory changes, crypt architecture, and microvascular patterns. CLE aids in targeted biopsy sampling, improves diagnostic accuracy, and provides valuable insights into disease activity in colitis.
- **Endoscopic Mucosal Resection (EMR):** EMR is a minimally invasive technique used to remove focal lesions or dysplastic areas in the colonic mucosa, particularly in cases of colitis-associated neoplasia. EMR facilitates en bloc resection of dysplastic lesions, reduces the risk of incomplete resection, and preserves colonic architecture in patients with colitis.

4. Therapeutic Endoscopy:

In addition to diagnostic evaluation, endoscopic interventions play a crucial role in the management of colitis, offering minimally invasive treatment options for mucosal healing, symptom control, and complication management. Therapeutic endoscopic procedures in colitis include:

- **Mucosal Healing:** Endoscopic therapy aims to achieve mucosal healing and resolution of inflammation in patients with colitis. Topical therapies, including 5-aminosalicylic acid (5-ASA) enemas or suppositories, rectal corticosteroids, and biologic agents, are administered via endoscopic route to target inflamed mucosa and induce remission.
- **Dilation:** Endoscopic balloon dilation is used to relieve colonic strictures and improve luminal patency in patients with inflammatory strictures or fibrotic changes associated with colitis. Dilation procedures may be performed under endoscopic guidance using controlled inflation of a balloon catheter, allowing gradual expansion of the narrowed colonic segment and restoration of bowel function.
- **Hemostasis:** Endoscopic hemostatic techniques are utilized to manage gastrointestinal bleeding in patients with colitis, including ulcers, erosions, or vascular lesions. Hemostatic modalities such as thermal coagulation, hemoclipping, or injection sclerotherapy are employed to achieve immediate control of bleeding and prevent further hemorrhage.
- **Stricture Management:** Endoscopic stricturoplasty or stent placement may be performed to alleviate symptoms and improve luminal patency in patients with colonic strictures refractory to medical therapy. Endoscopic dilation or placement of self-expanding metallic stents allows mechanical expansion of the narrowed segment, relieving obstruction and facilitating

passage of fecal contents.
- **Percutaneous Endoscopic Gastrostomy (PEG):** PEG tube placement may be indicated in patients with severe colitis or impaired oral intake requiring nutritional support. Endoscopic-guided placement of a PEG tube provides enteral access for feeding, medication administration, and decompression of the gastrointestinal tract, improving nutritional status and facilitating recovery.

5. Multimodal Imaging and Endoscopic Techniques:

Integration of multimodal imaging and advanced endoscopic techniques enhances diagnostic accuracy, enables targeted therapy, and improves outcomes in patients with colitis. Combining endoscopic findings with radiological imaging, molecular biomarkers, and histological evaluation allows comprehensive assessment of disease activity, identification of complications, and personalized treatment planning. Key advantages of multimodal imaging and endoscopic techniques in colitis include:

- **Precision Medicine:** Multimodal imaging and endoscopic techniques enable personalized treatment approaches tailored to individual patient characteristics, disease severity, and treatment response. Integration of clinical, endoscopic, and radiological data facilitates shared decision-making and optimization of therapeutic strategies in colitis management.
- **Real-Time Assessment:** Advanced endoscopic techniques provide real-time visualization and characterization of colonic mucosal changes, allowing immediate assessment of disease activity, severity, and response to therapy. Rapid evaluation of endoscopic findings guides treatment decisions and minimizes delays in therapeutic intervention, leading to improved

patient outcomes.
- **Early Detection of Complications:** Multimodal imaging facilitates early detection of colitis-related complications, including strictures, perforation, abscess formation, and dysplasia. Timely recognition of complications allows prompt intervention, reduces morbidity and mortality, and preserves colonic function in patients with colitis.
- **Optimization of Surveillance:** Integration of endoscopic surveillance protocols with advanced imaging techniques enhances detection of dysplasia and neoplastic changes in patients with colitis. Combined use of chromoendoscopy, high-definition imaging, and targeted biopsies improves diagnostic yield, reduces sampling errors, and enhances surveillance effectiveness in colitis-associated neoplasia.

Conclusion:

Endoscopic and imaging studies are indispensable tools in the diagnostic evaluation and management of colitis, offering precise visualization of colonic inflammation, mucosal changes, and associated complications. These diagnostic modalities enable accurate diagnosis, assessment of disease activity, and monitoring of treatment response in patients with colitis. Integration of multimodal imaging, advanced endoscopic techniques, and therapeutic interventions facilitates personalized treatment approaches, improves patient outcomes, and optimizes colitis management strategies. Collaborative efforts between gastroenterologists, radiologists, endoscopists, and other healthcare providers are essential for delivering comprehensive care and achieving therapeutic success in patients with colitis.

Histological Evaluation in Colitis: Unveiling Mucosal Changes and Disease Pathology

Histological evaluation plays a fundamental role in the diagnosis, characterization, and management of colitis, providing invaluable insights into the microscopic changes within the colonic mucosa. By examining tissue samples obtained via endoscopic biopsies or surgical resections, histopathologists can identify specific histological features indicative of colitis, assess disease severity, differentiate between different types of colitis, and detect complications such as dysplasia or malignancy. This comprehensive analysis aids in guiding treatment decisions, monitoring disease progression, and optimizing patient care. Here, we delve into the significance of histological evaluation in colitis, highlighting key histopathological findings and their clinical implications.

1. Microscopic Features of Colitis:

Histological examination of colonic mucosal biopsies allows visualization of characteristic microscopic features associated with colitis. These features include:

- **Inflammatory Infiltrate:** The presence of inflammatory infiltrate within the lamina propria is a hallmark feature of colitis. This infiltrate typically consists of lymphocytes, plasma cells, neutrophils, and eosinophils, reflecting the underlying immune-mediated inflammation.
- **Crypt Distortion:** Crypt distortion, characterized by irregular crypt architecture, branching, or dropout, is a common finding in colitis. Crypt distortion results from epithelial injury, inflammation, and regenerative changes, reflecting the dynamic nature of the disease

process.
- **Epithelial Injury:** Epithelial injury manifests as loss of surface epithelium, erosion, ulceration, or crypt abscess formation. These changes reflect mucosal damage and disruption of the epithelial barrier integrity, predisposing to bacterial translocation and inflammation.
- **Cryptitis and Crypt Abscesses:** Cryptitis, inflammation within colonic crypts, and crypt abscesses, collections of neutrophils within crypt lumina, are characteristic features of active colitis. These findings indicate ongoing mucosal inflammation and epithelial injury.
- **Architectural Changes:** Architectural changes such as crypt branching, distortion, or loss of crypt architecture may be observed in chronic colitis, reflecting long-standing inflammation and mucosal remodeling.
- **Lamina Propria Fibrosis:** Fibrosis of the lamina propria, characterized by collagen deposition and fibroblast proliferation, may occur in chronic colitis. Lamina propria fibrosis is associated with mucosal scarring, stricturing complications, and impaired mucosal healing.

2. Differentiating Types of Colitis:

Histological evaluation plays a crucial role in distinguishing between different types of colitis, including:

- **Ulcerative Colitis (UC):** Histological features of UC include diffuse inflammation, continuous mucosal involvement, crypt distortion, crypt abscesses, and absence of granulomas. The presence of pseudopolyps, crypt branching, and basal plasmacytosis may also support the diagnosis of UC.
- **Crohn's Disease (CD):** Histological findings in CD are heterogeneous and may include focal inflammation,

skip lesions, transmural involvement, non-caseating granulomas, and fissuring ulcers. The presence of granulomas, fissuring ulcers, and architectural distortion favor the diagnosis of CD.
- **Microscopic Colitis:** Microscopic colitis encompasses two subtypes, collagenous colitis and lymphocytic colitis, characterized by specific histological features. Collagenous colitis is defined by thickened subepithelial collagen band (>10 μm), while lymphocytic colitis is characterized by increased intraepithelial lymphocytes (>20 per 100 epithelial cells).
- **Ischemic Colitis:** Histological features of ischemic colitis include mucosal necrosis, submucosal hemorrhage, and inflammatory infiltrate, typically localized to the watershed areas of the colon. Ischemic colitis may exhibit a patchy distribution with segmental involvement.

3. Assessment of Disease Activity:

Histological evaluation provides valuable information about disease activity and severity in colitis, guiding treatment decisions and monitoring disease progression. Key histopathological parameters indicative of disease activity include:

- **Histological Activity Index:** Various scoring systems, such as the Geboes score for UC and the Crohn's Disease Endoscopic Index of Severity (CDEIS) for CD, quantify histological inflammation, architectural changes, and mucosal injury. These scoring systems facilitate standardized assessment of disease activity and treatment response.
- **Acute Inflammatory Changes:** Presence of acute inflammatory changes such as neutrophil infiltration, cryptitis, crypt abscesses, and epithelial injury indicates active disease activity in colitis. Evaluation of acute

inflammatory changes helps assess treatment response and guide therapeutic escalation.
- **Chronic Inflammatory Changes:** Chronic inflammatory changes such as lamina propria fibrosis, crypt distortion, and basal plasmacytosis indicate long-standing inflammation and tissue remodeling. Assessment of chronic inflammatory changes aids in prognostication and risk stratification in colitis.
- **Regenerative Changes:** Regenerative changes such as crypt hyperplasia, mucin depletion, and epithelial regeneration reflect the reparative response to mucosal injury and inflammation. Evaluation of regenerative changes provides insights into mucosal healing and treatment response in colitis.

4. Detection of Dysplasia and Neoplasia:

Histological evaluation plays a critical role in detecting dysplasia and neoplastic changes in patients with colitis, particularly those with long-standing disease or inflammatory bowel disease (IBD). Key considerations in the histological assessment of dysplasia and neoplasia include:

- **Dysplasia Grading:** Dysplasia is graded as low-grade or high-grade based on the degree of cytological and architectural abnormalities. Low-grade dysplasia (LGD) is characterized by mild to moderate cellular atypia, whereas high-grade dysplasia (HGD) exhibits severe cellular abnormalities and architectural disarray.
- **Dysplasia-associated Lesions or Masses (DALMs):** DALMs are focal lesions or polyps with dysplastic changes observed in patients with colitis, particularly UC. Histological evaluation of DALMs is essential for determining the presence and grade of dysplasia, guiding surveillance intervals, and informing therapeutic decisions.

- **Surveillance Biopsies:** Patients with colitis, particularly those with long-standing UC or CD involving the colon, require regular surveillance biopsies to detect dysplasia and neoplastic changes. Histological evaluation of surveillance biopsies helps identify dysplastic lesions at an early stage, enabling timely intervention and reducing the risk of colorectal cancer.

5. Therapeutic Response Assessment:

Histological evaluation is integral to assessing therapeutic response and monitoring disease activity in patients undergoing treatment for colitis. Key considerations in evaluating therapeutic response include:

- **Histological Remission:** Achievement of histological remission, defined by normalization of mucosal architecture, absence of acute inflammatory changes, and resolution of chronic inflammation, is a key treatment target in colitis management. Histological remission correlates with clinical remission and predicts favorable long-term outcomes in colitis.
- **Mucosal Healing:** Mucosal healing, characterized by restoration of mucosal integrity and absence of endoscopic or histological abnormalities, is associated with reduced risk of disease relapse, hospitalization, and colorectal cancer in colitis. Assessment of mucosal healing guides treatment escalation and optimization strategies in colitis management.
- **Response Assessment Tools:** Various histological scoring systems, such as the Robarts Histopathology Index (RHI) for UC and the Nancy Histological Index (NHI) for CD, facilitate standardized assessment of therapeutic response and disease activity in colitis. These scoring systems integrate histological parameters, including inflammation, regeneration, and architectural

changes, to quantify disease severity and treatment response objectively.

- **Biomarkers of Response:** Histological evaluation may include assessment of biomarkers associated with treatment response and prognosis in colitis. Biomarkers such as mucosal cytokine expression, immune cell infiltrates, and molecular signatures provide insights into disease pathogenesis, therapeutic targets, and predictive factors for treatment response.

6. Histological Challenges and Pitfalls:

Despite its utility, histological evaluation in colitis poses certain challenges and limitations that must be recognized and addressed:

- **Sampling Variability:** Histological interpretation may be influenced by sampling variability, as colonic inflammation and histological changes may exhibit patchy distribution. Adequate sampling from multiple colonic segments and representative biopsy sites is essential to minimize sampling bias and ensure accurate histological assessment.
- **Overlap with Normal Variants:** Histological features of colitis may overlap with normal variants or other non-inflammatory conditions, posing diagnostic challenges. Discriminating between inflammatory changes, reactive epithelial changes, and non-specific findings requires expertise and correlation with clinical and endoscopic findings.
- **Histological Mimics:** Certain conditions, such as infectious colitis, ischemic colitis, or drug-induced colitis, may mimic the histological features of inflammatory bowel disease (IBD). Histological evaluation should consider clinical context, microbiological testing, and medication history

to differentiate between inflammatory and non-inflammatory etiologies.
- **Dysplasia Detection:** Detection of dysplasia in colitis poses diagnostic challenges due to the presence of confounding inflammatory changes and reactive epithelial alterations. Histological interpretation of dysplasia requires meticulous examination, correlation with clinical risk factors, and consideration of ancillary techniques such as chromoendoscopy or molecular testing.

7. Future Directions in Histological Evaluation:

Advances in histological techniques and molecular profiling hold promise for enhancing diagnostic accuracy, predicting treatment response, and guiding personalized therapy in colitis. Future directions in histological evaluation include:

- **Digital Pathology:** Adoption of digital pathology platforms allows remote consultation, image analysis, and integration of artificial intelligence (AI) algorithms for automated histological assessment. Digital pathology enhances efficiency, standardization, and quality assurance in histological evaluation, facilitating collaborative research and clinical decision-making in colitis.
- **Molecular Profiling:** Integration of molecular profiling techniques, such as gene expression profiling, microbiome analysis, and proteomic profiling, provides deeper insights into disease pathogenesis, biomarker discovery, and therapeutic targets in colitis. Molecular signatures may aid in stratifying patients based on disease phenotype, predicting treatment response, and identifying novel therapeutic interventions.
- **Precision Medicine:** The era of precision medicine aims to individualize treatment strategies based on

patient-specific characteristics, including histological phenotype, genetic profile, and biomarker expression. Precision medicine approaches leverage histological evaluation, molecular testing, and clinical data to tailor personalized therapy and optimize outcomes in colitis management.

In conclusion, histological evaluation plays a pivotal role in the diagnosis, characterization, and management of colitis, offering valuable insights into mucosal changes, disease activity, and therapeutic response. Histopathological assessment enables differentiation between different types of colitis, detection of dysplasia and neoplasia, and monitoring of treatment efficacy. Continued advancements in histological techniques, molecular profiling, and precision medicine hold promise for improving diagnostic accuracy, prognostication, and therapeutic outcomes in colitis. Collaborative efforts between clinicians, pathologists, and researchers are essential for advancing our understanding of colitis pathophysiology and optimizing patient care in this complex disease.

CHAPTER 5: PATHOGENESIS OF COLITIS

Genetic Predisposition in Colitis: Unraveling the Role of Genetic Factors in Disease Susceptibility

Colitis, encompassing conditions such as ulcerative colitis (UC), Crohn's disease (CD), and other forms of inflammatory bowel disease (IBD), is characterized by chronic inflammation of the gastrointestinal tract. While environmental factors play a significant role in disease pathogenesis, genetic predisposition is increasingly recognized as a key determinant of susceptibility to colitis. Understanding the genetic basis of colitis provides valuable insights into disease etiology, pathophysiology, and personalized treatment approaches. In this section, we explore the genetic factors implicated in colitis susceptibility, highlighting key genes and pathways involved in disease development.

1. Familial Aggregation and Heritability:

The familial clustering of colitis cases underscores the importance of genetic predisposition in disease susceptibility. Studies have consistently demonstrated an increased risk of colitis among first-degree relatives of affected individuals, indicating a significant genetic component to disease pathogenesis. The heritability estimates for colitis range from 15% to 30%, emphasizing the substantial contribution of genetic factors to disease risk.

2. Genetic Variants Associated with Colitis:

Advances in genome-wide association studies (GWAS) and next-generation sequencing have led to the identification of numerous genetic variants associated with colitis susceptibility. Key genes and loci implicated in UC, CD, and IBD susceptibility include:

- **NOD2/CARD15:** Variants in the NOD2 gene, encoding a cytosolic pattern recognition receptor involved in innate immunity and bacterial sensing, are strongly associated with CD susceptibility. NOD2 variants confer increased risk of CD and influence disease phenotype, particularly ileal involvement and stricturing behavior.
- **IL23R:** Genetic variants in the IL23R gene, encoding the interleukin-23 receptor subunit, have been linked to both UC and CD susceptibility. IL23R variants modulate immune responses and Th17 cell differentiation, contributing to aberrant inflammatory signaling in colitis.
- **ATG16L1:** Variants in the autophagy-related 16-like 1 (ATG16L1) gene are associated with increased risk of CD and altered autophagy-mediated bacterial clearance in intestinal epithelial cells. ATG16L1 variants influence Paneth cell function, mucosal barrier integrity, and susceptibility to microbial dysbiosis in colitis.
- **IRGM:** The immunity-related GTPase M (IRGM) gene, involved in autophagy and intracellular pathogen clearance, harbors variants associated with CD susceptibility. IRGM polymorphisms modulate

antimicrobial responses, xenophagy, and epithelial barrier function in colitis.
- **HLA Complex:** Genetic variants within the major histocompatibility complex (MHC), particularly HLA-DQ and HLA-DR loci, confer susceptibility to UC and CD. HLA alleles influence antigen presentation, T cell activation, and adaptive immune responses in colitis pathogenesis.
- **IL10 and IL10RA:** Variants in the interleukin-10 (IL-10) gene and its receptor IL10RA are associated with early-onset and severe forms of IBD, including infantile-onset CD and UC. IL-10 signaling defects impair regulatory T cell function, immune tolerance, and mucosal homeostasis in colitis.

3. Polygenic Risk Scores (PRS) and Genetic Risk Profiling:

The cumulative effect of multiple genetic variants on colitis susceptibility is captured using polygenic risk scores (PRS), which integrate data from GWAS and genome-wide association meta-analyses. PRS analysis enables stratification of individuals based on their genetic risk profile and provides insights into disease susceptibility, severity, and treatment response. Genetic risk profiling may inform personalized risk assessment, screening protocols, and therapeutic decision-making in colitis management.

4. Gene-Environment Interactions:

Genetic predisposition to colitis interacts with environmental factors, including microbial triggers, dietary factors, smoking, and stress, to modulate disease risk and phenotype. Gene-environment interactions influence disease penetrance, clinical course, and treatment response in colitis. Understanding the interplay between genetic susceptibility and environmental exposures is crucial for unraveling disease pathogenesis and developing targeted interventions.

5. Pharmacogenomics and Personalized Therapy:

Genetic variants associated with drug metabolism, pharmacokinetics, and pharmacodynamics influence individual responses to colitis therapies, including immunomodulators, biologic agents, and thiopurines. Pharmacogenomic profiling enables personalized therapy selection, dosing optimization, and prediction of treatment outcomes in colitis patients. Tailoring treatment strategies based on genetic factors enhances therapeutic efficacy, minimizes adverse effects, and improves patient outcomes in colitis management.

In conclusion, genetic predisposition plays a significant role in colitis susceptibility, influencing disease risk, phenotype, and treatment response. Identification of key genetic variants and pathways associated with colitis susceptibility provides insights into disease pathogenesis and facilitates personalized approaches to therapy. Integration of genetic risk profiling, polygenic risk scores, and pharmacogenomics into clinical practice holds promise for optimizing patient care and advancing precision medicine in colitis management. Collaborative efforts between geneticists, gastroenterologists, and researchers are essential for translating genetic discoveries into clinical applications and improving outcomes for individuals affected by colitis.

Environmental Triggers in Colitis: Unraveling the Role of Extrinsic Factors in Disease Pathogenesis

Colitis, encompassing inflammatory bowel diseases (IBD) such as ulcerative colitis (UC), Crohn's disease (CD), and other forms of colitis, is characterized by chronic inflammation of the gastrointestinal tract. While genetic predisposition plays a significant role in disease susceptibility, environmental triggers are increasingly recognized as key contributors to disease onset, exacerbation, and progression. Understanding the environmental factors implicated in colitis pathogenesis is essential for elucidating disease mechanisms, identifying preventive strategies, and optimizing therapeutic interventions. In this section, we explore the diverse array of environmental triggers implicated in colitis development, highlighting their impact on disease susceptibility and clinical outcomes.

1. Microbial Dysbiosis:

Alterations in the composition, diversity, and function of the intestinal microbiota, termed microbial dysbiosis, have emerged as a central environmental factor in colitis pathogenesis. Dysbiotic microbiota are characterized by reduced microbial diversity, overgrowth of pathogenic bacteria, depletion of beneficial commensals, and disruption of microbial-host interactions. Key microbial triggers implicated in colitis include:

- **Pathogenic Bacteria:** Enteric pathogens such as Escherichia coli, Salmonella spp., Campylobacter spp., and Clostridium difficile can trigger acute infectious colitis or exacerbate chronic inflammatory responses in susceptible individuals. Pathogenic bacteria disrupt intestinal barrier function, induce mucosal inflammation, and promote dysbiosis through toxin production, epithelial invasion, and immune evasion mechanisms.
- **Dysbiotic Communities:** Dysbiosis of the gut microbiota, characterized by alterations in microbial composition, metabolic activity, and immunomodulatory potential, contributes to colitis pathogenesis. Dysbiotic communities are associated with reduced microbial diversity, expansion of pro-inflammatory taxa, and impaired barrier integrity, predisposing to mucosal inflammation and immune dysregulation in colitis.

- **Microbial Metabolites:** Microbial-derived metabolites, including short-chain fatty acids (SCFAs), bile acids, and trimethylamine-N-oxide (TMAO), modulate host immune responses, epithelial barrier function, and inflammatory signaling in colitis. Dysregulated production of microbial metabolites may promote mucosal inflammation, oxidative stress, and dysbiosis in colitis pathogenesis.

2. Dietary Factors:

Dietary factors play a crucial role in modulating gut microbiota composition, mucosal immune responses, and epithelial barrier function, thereby influencing colitis susceptibility and disease severity. Key dietary triggers implicated in colitis development include:

- **Western Diet:** High-fat, high-sugar Western diets rich in processed foods, red meat, and artificial additives are associated with increased risk of colitis and IBD exacerbations. Western diets promote dysbiosis, mucosal inflammation, and metabolic dysfunction through alterations in gut microbiota composition, nutrient availability, and inflammatory signaling pathways.
- **Fiber Deficiency:** Inadequate dietary fiber intake, characteristic of Western diets, compromises intestinal barrier function, microbial diversity, and mucosal immune homeostasis, predisposing to colitis development. Fiber deficiency impairs mucosal healing, exacerbates dysbiosis, and promotes pro-inflammatory signaling in the gut, contributing to mucosal inflammation and disease progression.
- **Food Additives:** Certain food additives, including emulsifiers, artificial sweeteners, and preservatives, disrupt gut microbiota composition, epithelial barrier integrity, and mucosal immune responses, exacerbating

colitis susceptibility and severity. Food additives promote dysbiosis, intestinal permeability, and mucosal inflammation through direct effects on microbial communities and host immune cells.

3. Lifestyle Factors:

Environmental lifestyle factors, including smoking, stress, medication use, and socioeconomic status, influence colitis susceptibility and disease outcomes. Key lifestyle triggers implicated in colitis pathogenesis include:

- **Smoking:** Cigarette smoking exhibits differential effects on UC and CD, with protective effects observed in UC and exacerbating effects observed in CD. Smoking modulates mucosal immune responses, microbial composition, and epithelial barrier function, contributing to disease heterogeneity and treatment response in colitis.
- **Stress and Psychosocial Factors:** Psychological stress, anxiety, and depression are associated with increased risk of colitis onset, exacerbation of symptoms, and disease relapse. Stress-induced alterations in neuroendocrine signaling, immune function, and gut-brain axis communication promote mucosal inflammation, dysbiosis, and barrier dysfunction in colitis.
- **Medication Use:** Certain medications, including nonsteroidal anti-inflammatory drugs (NSAIDs), antibiotics, proton pump inhibitors (PPIs), and oral contraceptives, may influence colitis susceptibility and disease outcomes. Medications alter gut microbiota composition, mucosal immunity, and epithelial barrier integrity, potentially exacerbating mucosal inflammation and dysbiosis in susceptible individuals.

4. Environmental Exposures:

Environmental exposures, including pollution, urbanization, hygiene practices, and occupational hazards, may influence colitis risk and disease outcomes. Key environmental triggers implicated in colitis development include:

- **Air Pollution:** Ambient air pollution, characterized by particulate matter (PM), ozone (O3), nitrogen dioxide (NO2), and sulfur dioxide (SO2), is associated with increased risk of colitis onset, exacerbation of symptoms, and disease progression. Air pollutants induce oxidative stress, inflammation, and mucosal barrier dysfunction, promoting immune-mediated colitis pathogenesis.
- **Urbanization and Hygiene Hypothesis:** Urbanization and Westernized lifestyles are associated with increased colitis prevalence, implicating environmental and lifestyle factors in disease susceptibility. The hygiene hypothesis posits that reduced microbial exposure, antibiotic use, and sanitation practices in urban environments disrupt immune tolerance mechanisms, predisposing to autoimmune and inflammatory disorders such as colitis.
- **Occupational Exposures:** Occupational exposures to environmental toxins, heavy metals, pesticides, and industrial chemicals may increase colitis risk and exacerbate disease severity. Occupational hazards disrupt intestinal barrier function, immune regulation, and microbial ecology, contributing to mucosal inflammation and dysbiosis in susceptible individuals.

5. Microbial-Environmental Interactions:

Interactions between microbial dysbiosis and environmental triggers play a critical role in colitis pathogenesis, shaping disease susceptibility, severity, and clinical outcomes. Microbial-environmental interactions modulate mucosal immune responses, barrier integrity, and inflammatory signaling, influencing disease heterogeneity and treatment response in colitis. Understanding the complex interplay between microbial dysbiosis, dietary factors, lifestyle triggers, and environmental exposures is essential for unraveling disease mechanisms and developing targeted interventions in colitis management.

In conclusion, environmental triggers play a multifaceted role in colitis pathogenesis, influencing disease susceptibility, severity, and clinical outcomes. Microbial dysbiosis, dietary factors, lifestyle triggers, and environmental exposures interact dynamically to modulate mucosal inflammation, dysbiosis, and immune dysregulation in colitis. Identifying and mitigating environmental triggers is crucial for preventing disease onset, optimizing therapeutic interventions, and improving outcomes in individuals affected by colitis. Collaborative efforts between clinicians, researchers, and policymakers are essential for addressing environmental determinants of colitis and advancing strategies for disease prevention and management.

Dysregulation of the Gut Microbiota in Colitis: Unveiling the Role of Microbial Imbalance in Disease Pathogenesis

Colitis, encompassing conditions such as ulcerative colitis (UC), Crohn's disease (CD), and other forms of inflammatory bowel disease (IBD), is characterized by chronic inflammation of the gastrointestinal tract. Among the multifactorial contributors to colitis pathogenesis, dysregulation of the gut microbiota has emerged as a central mechanism driving mucosal inflammation, immune dysregulation, and barrier dysfunction. Understanding the complex interplay between host-microbiota interactions, dysbiosis, and colitis pathogenesis is essential for elucidating disease mechanisms and developing targeted therapeutic strategies. In this section, we delve into the intricate relationship between dysregulation of the gut microbiota and colitis, exploring the key microbial alterations implicated in disease development and progression.

1. Microbial Dysbiosis in Colitis:

Microbial dysbiosis refers to the disruption of normal microbial composition, diversity, and function in the gut ecosystem, characterized by imbalances in beneficial commensals, pathogenic bacteria, and microbial metabolites. Dysbiosis of the gut microbiota is a hallmark feature of colitis, contributing to mucosal inflammation, immune dysregulation, and barrier dysfunction. Key microbial alterations associated with colitis include:

- **Reduced Microbial Diversity:** Colitis patients exhibit decreased microbial diversity and richness in the gut microbiota, characterized by loss of beneficial commensals and expansion of pathogenic bacteria. Reduced microbial diversity is associated with impaired mucosal resilience, dysregulated immune responses, and susceptibility to mucosal inflammation in colitis.
- **Expansion of Pathogenic Taxa:** Dysbiosis of the gut microbiota in colitis is characterized by expansion of pathogenic taxa such as Enterobacteriaceae, Fusobacterium spp., Proteobacteria, and adherent-invasive Escherichia coli (AIEC). Pathogenic bacteria promote mucosal inflammation, epithelial barrier dysfunction, and immune activation through toxin production, virulence factors, and inflammatory signaling pathways.
- **Disruption of Microbial Metabolism:** Dysregulation of microbial metabolism and metabolite production contributes to colitis pathogenesis, altering host-microbiota interactions, and immune homeostasis. Dysbiotic microbiota produce aberrant levels of short-chain fatty acids (SCFAs), bile acids, and secondary

metabolites, disrupting mucosal integrity, barrier function, and inflammatory signaling in colitis.
- **Loss of Butyrate-Producing Bacteria:** Butyrate-producing bacteria such as Faecalibacterium prausnitzii, Roseburia spp., and Eubacterium rectale are depleted in colitis patients, resulting in reduced butyrate production and impaired mucosal healing. Butyrate exerts anti-inflammatory, immunomodulatory, and barrier-stabilizing effects in the gut, protecting against mucosal inflammation and dysbiosis in colitis.

2. Host-Microbiota Interactions:

The gut microbiota interacts dynamically with host epithelial cells, immune cells, and mucosal factors to regulate intestinal homeostasis, immune tolerance, and barrier integrity. Dysregulated host-microbiota interactions contribute to colitis pathogenesis through:

- **Epithelial Barrier Dysfunction:** Dysbiotic microbiota disrupt epithelial barrier function, mucin production, and tight junction integrity, promoting translocation of luminal antigens and bacterial products into the lamina propria. Epithelial barrier dysfunction triggers mucosal inflammation, immune activation, and dysregulated host responses in colitis.
- **Immune Dysregulation:** Dysbiosis of the gut microbiota alters immune cell activation, cytokine production, and immune tolerance mechanisms in the intestinal mucosa, predisposing to exaggerated immune responses and chronic inflammation in colitis. Dysbiotic microbiota activate pro-inflammatory signaling pathways, recruit immune cells, and perturb regulatory T cell function, exacerbating mucosal inflammation in colitis.
- **Mucosal Inflammation:** Dysregulated host-microbiota interactions trigger mucosal inflammation,

characterized by infiltration of inflammatory cells, cytokine secretion, and tissue damage in the intestinal mucosa. Dysbiotic microbiota activate toll-like receptors (TLRs), nucleotide-binding oligomerization domain-like receptors (NLRs), and inflammasomes, inducing pro-inflammatory signaling cascades and perpetuating mucosal inflammation in colitis.

3. Impact of Dysbiosis on Disease Severity:

The severity and clinical course of colitis are influenced by the degree of microbial dysbiosis, with alterations in microbial composition, diversity, and function correlating with disease activity, treatment response, and prognosis. Dysbiosis of the gut microbiota is associated with increased disease severity, treatment resistance, and risk of complications in colitis patients. Key factors influencing the impact of dysbiosis on disease severity include:

- **Disease Phenotype:** The specific microbial alterations observed in colitis may vary based on disease phenotype, location, and severity. Patients with extensive colonic involvement or penetrating CD may exhibit distinct microbial profiles compared to those with limited disease extent or inflammatory UC.
- **Treatment Response:** Microbial dysbiosis may influence treatment response and therapeutic outcomes in colitis patients, with alterations in microbial composition predicting response to pharmacological interventions, dietary modifications, or fecal microbiota transplantation (FMT). Restoration of eubiosis and normalization of microbial diversity may enhance treatment efficacy and improve clinical outcomes in colitis management.
- **Complications and Progression:** Dysbiosis of the gut microbiota is associated with increased risk of colitis-

related complications, including strictures, fistulas, abscesses, and colorectal cancer. Dysbiotic microbiota promote mucosal damage, dysplasia, and neoplastic transformation, accelerating disease progression and increasing the burden of morbidity and mortality in colitis patients.

4. Therapeutic Strategies Targeting Dysbiosis:

Therapeutic interventions aimed at modulating the gut microbiota represent promising strategies for mitigating dysbiosis, restoring microbial balance, and improving clinical outcomes in colitis patients. Key therapeutic approaches targeting dysbiosis in colitis include:

- **Probiotics and Prebiotics:** Administration of probiotics, live microbial supplements with beneficial effects on host health, and prebiotics, dietary substrates that promote the growth of beneficial commensals, may modulate the gut microbiota and ameliorate mucosal inflammation in colitis. Probiotics such as Lactobacillus spp., Bifidobacterium spp., and Saccharomyces boulardii exhibit anti-inflammatory, immunomodulatory, and barrier-stabilizing effects in colitis management.
- **Dietary Modifications:** Dietary interventions targeting microbial dysbiosis, such as high-fiber diets, Mediterranean diets, and low-fermentable oligosaccharide, disaccharide, monosaccharide, and polyol (FODMAP) diets, may promote eubiosis and mitigate mucosal inflammation in colitis. Dietary modifications alter microbial composition, metabolite production, and mucosal immune responses, influencing disease activity and treatment response in colitis patients.
- **Fecal Microbiota Transplantation (FMT):** FMT involves the transfer of fecal microbial communities from

healthy donors to colitis patients, aiming to restore microbial balance, diversify microbial ecology, and alleviate mucosal inflammation. FMT is emerging as a promising therapeutic approach for refractory colitis cases, particularly recurrent Clostridium difficile infection (CDI) and steroid-resistant IBD. FMT restores microbial diversity, enhances mucosal healing, and modulates immune responses in colitis patients, leading to improved clinical outcomes and reduced disease recurrence rates.

- **Antibiotics and Microbial Targeted Therapies:** Antibiotics targeting specific pathogenic bacteria or dysbiotic microbial communities may modulate gut microbiota composition and alleviate mucosal inflammation in colitis. Antibiotics such as metronidazole, ciprofloxacin, and rifaximin are used to treat active colitis flares, infectious exacerbations, or dysbiotic microbial overgrowth in colitis patients.
- **Microbial Modulators:** Microbial modulators, including antibiotics, probiotics, and microbial metabolites, may modulate gut microbiota composition, diversity, and function in colitis. Microbial modulators exert anti-inflammatory, immunomodulatory, and barrier-stabilizing effects in the intestinal mucosa, mitigating mucosal inflammation and dysbiosis in colitis management.

5. Future Directions in Microbiota-Based Therapies:

Advances in microbiota-based therapies hold promise for precision medicine approaches in colitis management, aiming to restore microbial balance, personalize therapeutic interventions, and optimize clinical outcomes. Future directions in microbiota-based therapies include:

- **Microbiota Profiling:** Comprehensive profiling of the

gut microbiota using next-generation sequencing, metagenomic analysis, and multi-omics approaches enables characterization of microbial composition, functional potential, and metabolic activity in colitis. Microbiota profiling facilitates personalized risk assessment, treatment selection, and monitoring of therapeutic response in colitis patients.

- **Microbial Therapeutics:** Development of microbial therapeutics, including live biotherapeutic products (LBPs), engineered probiotics, and microbial consortia, offers targeted interventions for modulating gut microbiota composition and function in colitis. Microbial therapeutics deliver specific microbial strains, metabolites, or bioactive compounds to the intestinal mucosa, restoring eubiosis and ameliorating mucosal inflammation in colitis management.
- **Microbiota Engineering:** Engineering of the gut microbiota using synthetic biology, CRISPR-Cas gene editing, and microbial consortia design enables manipulation of microbial composition, function, and interactions in colitis. Microbiota engineering strategies target dysbiotic microbial communities, enhance microbial diversity, and promote mucosal homeostasis in colitis patients, offering potential avenues for disease modification and remission induction.
- **Personalized Microbiome Medicine:** Integration of microbiome data with clinical phenotypes, genetic profiles, and environmental exposures enables personalized microbiome medicine approaches in colitis management. Personalized microbiome medicine leverages microbiota profiling, host-microbiota interactions, and therapeutic interventions to tailor precision therapies, optimize treatment outcomes, and improve patient care in colitis.

In conclusion, dysregulation of the gut microbiota plays

a pivotal role in colitis pathogenesis, influencing disease susceptibility, severity, and treatment response. Understanding the complex interplay between host-microbiota interactions, dysbiosis, and colitis pathophysiology is essential for developing microbiota-based therapies, precision medicine approaches, and targeted interventions in colitis management. Continued advancements in microbiome research, microbial therapeutics, and personalized medicine hold promise for optimizing clinical outcomes and improving quality of life for individuals affected by colitis. Collaborative efforts between clinicians, researchers, and industry partners are essential for translating microbiome discoveries into innovative therapies and transformative solutions for colitis patients.

Immune Dysregulation and Inflammation in Colitis: Unraveling the Complex Interplay Between Host Immune Responses and Mucosal Inflammation

Colitis, encompassing conditions such as ulcerative colitis (UC), Crohn's disease (CD), and other forms of inflammatory bowel disease (IBD), is characterized by dysregulated immune responses and chronic inflammation of the gastrointestinal tract. Immune dysregulation and mucosal inflammation play pivotal roles in colitis pathogenesis, driving tissue damage, barrier dysfunction, and clinical manifestations of the disease. Understanding the intricate interplay between host immune cells, inflammatory mediators, and mucosal tissues is essential for elucidating disease mechanisms and developing targeted therapeutic strategies. In this section, we explore the multifaceted aspects of immune dysregulation and inflammation in colitis, highlighting key immune pathways, cytokines, and cellular interactions implicated in disease pathophysiology.

1. Innate Immune Responses:

Innate immune cells, including macrophages, dendritic cells, neutrophils, and innate lymphoid cells (ILCs), play crucial roles in sensing microbial pathogens, initiating inflammatory responses, and orchestrating mucosal immunity in colitis. Dysregulated innate immune responses contribute to mucosal inflammation, tissue damage, and barrier dysfunction in colitis through:

- **Macrophage Activation:** Dysfunctional macrophages exhibit aberrant activation states, polarization phenotypes, and cytokine profiles in colitis, promoting tissue injury, fibrosis, and granuloma formation. M1-polarized macrophages produce pro-inflammatory cytokines such as tumor necrosis factor-alpha (TNF-α), interleukin-1β (IL-1β), and interleukin-6 (IL-6), exacerbating mucosal inflammation and immune dysregulation in colitis.
- **Dendritic Cell Function:** Dendritic cells (DCs) are central mediators of antigen presentation, T cell activation, and immune tolerance in the intestinal mucosa. Dysregulated DC function in colitis results in impaired antigen presentation, T cell priming, and regulatory T cell (Treg) induction, leading to exaggerated immune responses and mucosal inflammation.
- **Neutrophil Infiltration:** Neutrophils are recruited to the inflamed mucosa in colitis, where they release reactive oxygen species (ROS), proteases, and pro-inflammatory cytokines, exacerbating tissue damage and inflammation. Dysregulated neutrophil recruitment, activation, and survival contribute to mucosal injury, epithelial barrier dysfunction, and clinical symptoms of colitis.
- **Innate Lymphoid Cells:** Innate lymphoid cells (ILCs),

including natural killer (NK) cells, group 1 ILCs (ILC1s), group 2 ILCs (ILC2s), and group 3 ILCs (ILC3s), modulate mucosal inflammation, barrier integrity, and tissue repair in colitis. Dysregulated ILC responses contribute to altered cytokine production, tissue fibrosis, and dysbiosis in colitis pathogenesis.

2. Adaptive Immune Responses:

Adaptive immune cells, including T cells, B cells, and antigen-presenting cells (APCs), mediate antigen-specific immune responses, antibody production, and immune memory in colitis. Dysregulated adaptive immune responses drive mucosal inflammation, autoimmunity, and tissue destruction in colitis through:

- **T Cell Activation:** Dysfunctional T cell subsets, including CD4+ T helper (Th) cells, CD8+ cytotoxic T cells, and regulatory T cells (Tregs), contribute to mucosal inflammation and immune dysregulation in colitis. Th1 and Th17 cells produce pro-inflammatory cytokines such as interferon-gamma (IFN-γ), interleukin-17 (IL-17), and interleukin-23 (IL-23), promoting epithelial barrier dysfunction and tissue damage in colitis.
- **B Cell Responses:** B cells play dual roles in colitis pathogenesis, producing pro-inflammatory antibodies and regulatory cytokines that modulate mucosal immunity and tissue repair. Dysregulated B cell activation, antibody production, and immune complex formation contribute to mucosal inflammation, autoantibody production, and immune complex-mediated tissue damage in colitis.
- **Antigen-Presenting Cells:** Dendritic cells, macrophages, and B cells serve as antigen-presenting cells (APCs) that initiate and regulate adaptive immune responses in colitis. Dysregulated APC function results in

altered antigen presentation, T cell activation, and immune tolerance mechanisms, exacerbating mucosal inflammation and immune dysregulation in colitis.

3. Cytokine Imbalance:

Cytokines orchestrate immune responses, inflammatory signaling, and tissue repair processes in the intestinal mucosa, influencing disease pathogenesis and clinical outcomes in colitis. Dysregulated cytokine production, signaling, and receptor activation contribute to mucosal inflammation, tissue damage, and clinical manifestations of colitis through:

- **Pro-Inflammatory Cytokines:** Pro-inflammatory cytokines, including TNF-α, IL-1β, IL-6, IL-12, IL-17, and IL-23, drive mucosal inflammation, immune cell activation, and tissue destruction in colitis. Dysregulated production of pro-inflammatory cytokines amplifies immune responses, perpetuates mucosal inflammation, and exacerbates disease severity in colitis.
- **Anti-Inflammatory Cytokines:** Anti-inflammatory cytokines, such as interleukin-10 (IL-10) and transforming growth factor-beta (TGF-β), regulate immune tolerance, mucosal healing, and tissue repair processes in the intestinal mucosa. Dysregulated production of anti-inflammatory cytokines impairs immune regulation, compromises mucosal healing, and exacerbates chronic inflammation in colitis.
- **Th17/Treg Imbalance:** Imbalance between Th17 and Treg cell subsets, characterized by increased Th17 cell activation and reduced Treg cell function, contributes to mucosal inflammation and immune dysregulation in colitis. Dysregulated Th17/Treg balance disrupts immune homeostasis, exacerbates autoimmunity, and promotes chronic inflammation in colitis pathogenesis.

4. Mucosal Inflammatory Pathways:

Inflammatory signaling pathways, including nuclear factor-kappa B (NF-κB), mitogen-activated protein kinase (MAPK), and Janus kinase-signal transducer and activator of transcription (JAK-STAT) pathways, mediate immune responses, cytokine production, and tissue damage in colitis. Dysregulated activation of mucosal inflammatory pathways perpetuates mucosal inflammation, barrier dysfunction, and clinical symptoms of colitis through:

- **NF-κB Signaling:** Dysregulated NF-κB signaling promotes immune cell activation, cytokine production, and inflammatory gene expression in the intestinal mucosa, amplifying mucosal inflammation and tissue damage in colitis. NF-κB inhibitors and anti-inflammatory agents targeting NF-κB signaling pathways may mitigate mucosal inflammation and improve clinical outcomes in colitis management.
- **MAPK Signaling:** Dysregulated MAPK signaling pathways, including extracellular signal-regulated kinase (ERK), c-Jun N-terminal kinase (JNK), and p38 MAPK, mediate inflammatory responses, cell proliferation, and apoptosis in the intestinal mucosa. Dysregulated MAPK activation exacerbates mucosal inflammation, epithelial barrier dysfunction, and tissue damage in colitis, perpetuating disease pathogenesis and clinical symptoms. Inhibition of MAPK signaling pathways using pharmacological inhibitors or targeted therapeutics may attenuate mucosal inflammation and improve outcomes in colitis patients.
- **JAK-STAT Signaling:** Dysregulated JAK-STAT signaling pathways modulate immune cell activation, cytokine receptor signaling, and inflammatory gene expression in the intestinal mucosa. Aberrant activation of JAK-STAT pathways promotes mucosal inflammation, immune dysregulation, and tissue damage in colitis.

JAK inhibitors and biologic therapies targeting cytokine receptors or downstream signaling molecules may mitigate inflammatory responses and ameliorate disease severity in colitis management.

5. Cellular Mediators of Inflammation:

Cellular mediators, including immune cells, epithelial cells, and stromal cells, play critical roles in orchestrating mucosal inflammation, tissue repair, and barrier maintenance in colitis. Dysregulated cellular responses contribute to mucosal inflammation, epithelial barrier dysfunction, and clinical manifestations of colitis through:

- **Immune Cell Infiltration:** Infiltration of immune cells, including T cells, B cells, macrophages, neutrophils, and eosinophils, into the intestinal mucosa drives mucosal inflammation, cytokine production, and tissue damage in colitis. Dysregulated immune cell recruitment, activation, and effector functions exacerbate mucosal inflammation and perpetuate chronic inflammation in colitis pathogenesis.
- **Epithelial Barrier Dysfunction:** Dysfunctional epithelial cells exhibit impaired barrier integrity, mucin production, and tight junction protein expression in the inflamed mucosa of colitis patients. Epithelial barrier dysfunction predisposes to microbial translocation, immune activation, and mucosal inflammation in colitis, perpetuating tissue damage and disease progression.
- **Stromal Cell Activation:** Intestinal stromal cells, including fibroblasts, myofibroblasts, and mesenchymal stem cells (MSCs), contribute to mucosal inflammation, tissue remodeling, and fibrosis in colitis. Dysregulated stromal cell activation promotes extracellular matrix deposition, tissue fibrosis, and stricture formation in the inflamed mucosa of colitis patients.

6. Therapeutic Strategies Targeting Immune Dysregulation:

Therapeutic interventions aimed at modulating immune dysregulation and inflammation represent cornerstone approaches in colitis management, aiming to alleviate mucosal inflammation, promote tissue repair, and improve clinical outcomes. Key therapeutic strategies targeting immune dysregulation in colitis include:

- **Immunomodulatory Agents:** Immunomodulatory agents, including corticosteroids, immunosuppressants, and biologic therapies, modulate immune responses, cytokine production, and inflammatory signaling pathways in the intestinal mucosa. Immunomodulatory agents attenuate mucosal inflammation, induce clinical remission, and reduce the risk of disease relapse in colitis patients.
- **Biologic Therapies:** Biologic therapies targeting specific cytokines, immune cells, or inflammatory mediators offer targeted interventions for modulating immune dysregulation and mucosal inflammation in colitis. Biologic therapies such as anti-TNF agents, anti-integrin antibodies, and anti-IL-12/IL-23 antibodies inhibit inflammatory pathways, suppress immune responses, and promote mucosal healing in colitis management.
- **Cell-Based Therapies:** Cell-based therapies, including mesenchymal stem cell (MSC) transplantation, regulatory T cell (Treg) infusion, and hematopoietic stem cell transplantation (HSCT), harness the immunomodulatory properties of stem cells or regulatory cells to modulate immune dysregulation and promote tissue repair in colitis. Cell-based therapies offer regenerative potential, immune tolerance induction, and disease-modifying effects in refractory colitis cases.
- **Targeted Immunotherapies:** Targeted

immunotherapies, including JAK inhibitors, cytokine receptor antagonists, and toll-like receptor (TLR) agonists, selectively modulate immune responses, inflammatory signaling, and mucosal inflammation in colitis. Targeted immunotherapies exhibit specificity for key immune pathways, cytokine receptors, or inflammatory mediators implicated in colitis pathogenesis, offering precision interventions for immune-mediated disease processes.

7. Future Directions in Immune Modulation:

Advances in immune modulation hold promise for precision medicine approaches in colitis management, aiming to personalize therapeutic interventions, optimize treatment outcomes, and minimize adverse effects. Future directions in immune modulation include:

- **Precision Medicine Approaches:** Integration of immunophenotyping, genetic profiling, and biomarker analysis enables personalized medicine approaches in colitis management, tailoring therapeutic interventions to individual patient characteristics, disease phenotypes, and treatment responses. Precision medicine approaches optimize treatment efficacy, minimize adverse effects, and improve outcomes in colitis patients.
- **Novel Immunotherapies:** Development of novel immunotherapies targeting emerging immune pathways, inflammatory mediators, or cellular targets offers innovative strategies for immune modulation in colitis. Novel immunotherapies may include small molecule inhibitors, monoclonal antibodies, engineered cell therapies, or gene editing techniques, aiming to precisely modulate immune responses and mucosal inflammation in colitis management.
- **Combination Therapies:** Combination therapies

targeting multiple immune pathways, cytokine networks, or cellular mediators offer synergistic effects and enhanced therapeutic efficacy in colitis management. Combination therapies may include dual immunomodulatory agents, biologic-immunosuppressant combinations, or sequential treatment regimens, aiming to optimize immune modulation and improve clinical outcomes in colitis patients.

- **Microbiota-Immune Interactions:** Integration of microbiome data with immune profiling enables characterization of microbiota-immune interactions, mucosal immune responses, and disease pathogenesis in colitis. Microbiota-immune interactions influence disease susceptibility, treatment response, and prognosis in colitis, offering potential targets for immune modulation and therapeutic intervention.

In conclusion, immune dysregulation and inflammation play pivotal roles in colitis pathogenesis, driving mucosal inflammation, tissue damage, and clinical manifestations of the disease. Understanding the complex interplay between host immune responses, inflammatory mediators, and mucosal tissues is essential for developing targeted therapeutic strategies, precision medicine approaches, and innovative interventions in colitis management. Continued advancements in immune modulation hold promise for optimizing treatment outcomes, improving quality of life, and achieving long-term remission in individuals affected by colitis. Collaborative efforts between clinicians, researchers, and industry partners are essential for translating immunological discoveries into transformative solutions for colitis patients.

Role of Oxidative Stress and Free Radicals in Colitis:

Unraveling the Molecular Mechanisms of Tissue Damage and Inflammation

Oxidative stress, characterized by an imbalance between reactive oxygen species (ROS) production and antioxidant defenses, plays a pivotal role in the pathogenesis of colitis. Inflammatory bowel diseases (IBD), including ulcerative colitis (UC) and Crohn's disease (CD), are associated with increased oxidative stress in the intestinal mucosa, leading to tissue damage, barrier dysfunction, and chronic inflammation. In this section, we delve into the intricate mechanisms by which oxidative stress and free radicals contribute to colitis pathophysiology, highlighting their impact on mucosal integrity, immune responses, and disease progression.

1. ROS Generation and Sources:

Reactive oxygen species (ROS), including superoxide anion (O_2^-), hydrogen peroxide (H_2O_2), hydroxyl radical ($\cdot OH$), and peroxynitrite ($ONOO^-$), are highly reactive molecules generated as byproducts of cellular metabolism and immune responses. In colitis, excessive ROS production occurs due to dysregulated inflammatory signaling, mitochondrial dysfunction, and oxidative burst reactions in immune cells. Major sources of ROS generation in colitis include:

- **Phagocytic Cells:** Neutrophils, macrophages, and dendritic cells generate ROS through the respiratory burst pathway during phagocytosis and immune responses. Excessive ROS production by activated phagocytic cells contributes to mucosal inflammation, tissue damage, and oxidative stress in colitis.
- **Mitochondria:** Mitochondrial dysfunction and electron transport chain (ETC) impairment lead to increased ROS production in colitis. Dysregulated mitochondrial metabolism, oxidative phosphorylation, and ATP production result in mitochondrial ROS generation,

exacerbating mucosal inflammation and cellular damage in colitis.

- **NADPH Oxidases:** NADPH oxidases (NOX), including NOX1, NOX2, and NOX4 isoforms, are membrane-bound enzymes that generate ROS as part of cellular signaling and host defense mechanisms. Dysregulated NOX activity and expression contribute to mucosal oxidative stress, immune dysregulation, and barrier dysfunction in colitis.
- **Inflammatory Signaling Pathways:** Dysregulated inflammatory signaling pathways, including nuclear factor-kappa B (NF-κB), mitogen-activated protein kinase (MAPK), and toll-like receptor (TLR) pathways, promote ROS production and oxidative stress in colitis. Inflammatory cytokines, such as tumor necrosis factor-alpha (TNF-α) and interleukin-1β (IL-1β), stimulate ROS generation through activation of NADPH oxidases and mitochondrial pathways.

2. Molecular Targets of Oxidative Damage:

Oxidative stress in colitis targets various molecular components of the intestinal mucosa, including lipids, proteins, nucleic acids, and cellular membranes. ROS-induced oxidative damage disrupts cellular homeostasis, impairs tissue repair mechanisms, and exacerbates mucosal inflammation in colitis through:

- **Lipid Peroxidation:** ROS-mediated lipid peroxidation leads to the generation of lipid peroxides, reactive aldehydes, and oxidative byproducts that damage cellular membranes and lipoproteins in the intestinal mucosa. Lipid peroxidation products, such as malondialdehyde (MDA) and 4-hydroxynonenal (4-HNE), trigger inflammatory responses, oxidative stress, and tissue injury in colitis.

- **Protein Oxidation:** ROS-induced protein oxidation results in the formation of protein carbonyl groups, oxidized amino acids, and protein adducts that alter protein structure, function, and stability in the intestinal mucosa. Protein oxidation compromises enzymatic activities, signaling pathways, and immune responses, exacerbating mucosal inflammation and tissue damage in colitis.
- **DNA Damage:** ROS-induced DNA damage, including oxidative base modifications, DNA strand breaks, and DNA adduct formation, disrupts genomic integrity and cellular function in the intestinal epithelium. DNA damage triggers cellular senescence, apoptosis, and mutagenesis, contributing to mucosal inflammation, dysplasia, and colorectal carcinogenesis in colitis.
- **Antioxidant Depletion:** Oxidative stress depletes antioxidant defenses, including enzymatic antioxidants (e.g., superoxide dismutase, catalase, glutathione peroxidase) and non-enzymatic antioxidants (e.g., glutathione, vitamins C and E), in the intestinal mucosa of colitis patients. Antioxidant depletion exacerbates ROS-induced oxidative damage, impairs cellular detoxification pathways, and perpetuates mucosal inflammation in colitis.

3. Oxidative Stress and Barrier Dysfunction:

Oxidative stress disrupts epithelial barrier function, mucin production, and tight junction integrity in the intestinal mucosa, leading to increased permeability, bacterial translocation, and immune activation in colitis. ROS-induced barrier dysfunction exacerbates mucosal inflammation, tissue damage, and disease progression through:

- **Tight Junction Disruption:** ROS-mediated oxidative modification of tight junction proteins, including

occludin, claudins, and zonula occludens (ZO), impairs intercellular junctional complexes and tight junction integrity in the intestinal epithelium. Tight junction disruption increases paracellular permeability, epithelial leakage, and bacterial translocation in colitis.
- **Mucin Degradation:** ROS-induced oxidative damage to mucin glycoproteins, such as MUC2, compromises mucus layer integrity, viscoelastic properties, and barrier function in the intestinal mucosa. Mucin degradation reduces mucus layer thickness, impairs bacterial clearance, and exacerbates mucosal inflammation in colitis.
- **Epithelial Cell Apoptosis:** ROS-induced oxidative stress triggers epithelial cell apoptosis, anoikis, and shedding in the intestinal mucosa of colitis patients. Epithelial cell loss disrupts epithelial barrier integrity, compromises mucosal defense mechanisms, and exacerbates mucosal inflammation in colitis pathogenesis.

4. ROS-Mediated Immune Dysregulation:

Oxidative stress modulates immune responses, inflammatory signaling, and immune cell functions in the intestinal mucosa, contributing to immune dysregulation and chronic inflammation in colitis. ROS-mediated immune dysregulation exacerbates mucosal inflammation, tissue damage, and disease severity through:

- **Immune Cell Activation:** ROS promote immune cell activation, cytokine production, and inflammatory mediator release in the intestinal mucosa of colitis patients. ROS activate signaling pathways, such as NF-κB and MAPK, in immune cells, amplifying inflammatory responses and exacerbating mucosal inflammation in colitis.
- **Cytokine Imbalance:** ROS modulate cytokine

production, signaling, and receptor activation in immune cells, altering the balance between pro-inflammatory and anti-inflammatory cytokines in the intestinal mucosa. ROS induce pro-inflammatory cytokines, such as TNF-α, IL-1β, and IL-6, while inhibiting anti-inflammatory cytokines, such as IL-10 and TGF-β, exacerbating mucosal inflammation in colitis.

- **Immune Cell Dysfunction:** ROS-induced oxidative stress impairs immune cell functions, including phagocytosis, antigen presentation, and regulatory T cell (Treg) differentiation, in the intestinal mucosa of colitis patients. Immune cell dysfunction compromises host defense mechanisms, immune tolerance induction, and regulatory responses, exacerbating mucosal inflammation and tissue damage in colitis pathogenesis.

5. Redox Signaling Pathways:

Redox signaling pathways regulate cellular responses to oxidative stress, inflammatory stimuli, and environmental cues in the intestinal mucosa, modulating immune activation, cytokine production, and tissue repair processes in colitis. Redox signaling pathways play dual roles in colitis pathophysiology, exerting pro-inflammatory and anti-inflammatory effects through:

- **Nuclear Factor-kappa B (NF-κB):** NF-κB is a key transcription factor that regulates inflammatory gene expression, immune cell activation, and oxidative stress responses in the intestinal mucosa. ROS-mediated activation of NF-κB signaling promotes inflammatory cytokine production, leukocyte recruitment, and mucosal inflammation in colitis.
- **Nrf2-Keap1 Pathway:** The nuclear factor erythroid 2-related factor 2 (Nrf2)-Kelch-like ECH-associated protein 1 (Keap1) pathway is a critical antioxidant defense

mechanism that regulates cellular responses to oxidative stress and xenobiotic exposure. Nrf2 activation induces antioxidant gene expression, detoxification pathways, and cytoprotective responses, mitigating oxidative stress and inflammation in colitis.
- **MAPK Signaling:** Mitogen-activated protein kinase (MAPK) signaling pathways, including extracellular signal-regulated kinase (ERK), c-Jun N-terminal kinase (JNK), and p38 MAPK, mediate cellular responses to oxidative stress, inflammatory cytokines, and growth factors in the intestinal mucosa. ROS-induced MAPK activation regulates immune cell functions, cytokine production, and tissue remodeling processes in colitis.
- **PI3K-Akt Pathway:** The phosphoinositide 3-kinase (PI3K)-Akt pathway modulates cellular survival, proliferation, and metabolism in response to growth factors, cytokines, and oxidative stress in the intestinal mucosa. ROS-mediated activation of the PI3K-Akt pathway promotes cell survival, epithelial repair, and mucosal regeneration in colitis.

6. Therapeutic Targeting of Oxidative Stress:

Therapeutic interventions targeting oxidative stress aim to mitigate ROS production, enhance antioxidant defenses, and restore redox balance in the intestinal mucosa of colitis patients. Strategies for therapeutic targeting of oxidative stress in colitis include:

- **Antioxidant Supplementation:** Antioxidant supplementation with vitamins C and E, glutathione precursors, polyphenols, and flavonoids scavenges ROS, neutralizes oxidative byproducts, and enhances antioxidant defenses in the intestinal mucosa. Antioxidant supplementation reduces mucosal inflammation, oxidative stress, and disease severity in

colitis patients.
- **Nrf2 Activators:** Pharmacological activators of the Nrf2-Keap1 pathway, such as sulforaphane, bardoxolone methyl, and dimethyl fumarate, induce antioxidant gene expression, detoxification pathways, and cytoprotective responses in the intestinal mucosa. Nrf2 activators enhance mucosal antioxidant defenses, mitigate oxidative stress, and ameliorate mucosal inflammation in colitis.
- **ROS Scavengers:** ROS scavengers, including superoxide dismutase (SOD) mimetics, catalase mimetics, and metal chelators, neutralize ROS, inhibit oxidative reactions, and mitigate tissue damage in the intestinal mucosa of colitis patients. ROS scavengers attenuate mucosal inflammation, oxidative stress, and barrier dysfunction in colitis management.
- **Inhibitors of ROS Production:** Pharmacological inhibitors of ROS-generating enzymes, such as NADPH oxidases, xanthine oxidase, and mitochondrial respiratory chain complexes, suppress ROS production, oxidative stress, and inflammatory responses in the intestinal mucosa. Inhibitors of ROS production reduce mucosal inflammation, tissue damage, and disease progression in colitis.
- **Redox-Active Compounds:** Redox-active compounds, including thiol compounds, metalloporphyrins, and redox-modulating agents, modulate cellular redox status, redox signaling pathways, and oxidative stress responses in the intestinal mucosa of colitis patients. Redox-active compounds restore redox balance, mitigate mucosal inflammation, and promote tissue repair in colitis management.

7. Future Directions in Oxidative Stress Research:

Advances in oxidative stress research hold promise for

developing innovative therapies, biomarkers, and diagnostic tools for colitis management, aiming to optimize treatment outcomes and improve patient care. Future directions in oxidative stress research include:

- **Precision Medicine Approaches:** Integration of oxidative stress biomarkers, redox profiles, and genetic variants enables personalized medicine approaches in colitis management, tailoring therapeutic interventions to individual patient characteristics, disease phenotypes, and treatment responses. Precision medicine approaches optimize treatment efficacy, minimize adverse effects, and improve outcomes in colitis patients.
- **Novel Redox-Targeted Therapies:** Development of novel redox-targeted therapies, including ROS scavengers, antioxidant enzymes, and redox-modulating agents, offers innovative strategies for mitigating oxidative stress and inflammation in colitis. Novel redox-targeted therapies may include gene therapy approaches, nanomedicine formulations, or targeted drug delivery systems, aiming to enhance therapeutic efficacy and reduce off-target effects in colitis management.
- **Redox Imaging Technologies:** Advancements in redox imaging technologies, such as fluorescence microscopy, magnetic resonance imaging (MRI), and positron emission tomography (PET), enable non-invasive assessment of oxidative stress, redox status, and tissue damage in the intestinal mucosa of colitis patients. Redox imaging technologies facilitate early detection of mucosal inflammation, monitoring of therapeutic response, and prediction of disease progression in colitis management.
- **Nutritional Interventions:** Dietary interventions targeting oxidative stress, such as antioxidant-rich diets, polyphenol supplementation, and omega-3 fatty

acids, may modulate mucosal redox balance, immune responses, and gut microbiota composition in colitis. Nutritional interventions offer adjunctive strategies for managing oxidative stress and inflammation in colitis patients, promoting mucosal healing and disease remission.

In conclusion, oxidative stress plays a central role in colitis pathogenesis, driving mucosal inflammation, tissue damage, and disease progression. Understanding the molecular mechanisms of oxidative stress, redox signaling pathways, and antioxidant defenses in the intestinal mucosa is essential for developing targeted therapeutic strategies, precision medicine approaches, and innovative interventions in colitis management. Continued advancements in oxidative stress research hold promise for optimizing treatment outcomes, improving quality of life, and achieving long-term remission in individuals affected by colitis. Collaborative efforts between clinicians, researchers, and industry partners are essential for translating oxidative stress discoveries into transformative solutions for colitis patients.

CHAPTER 6: TREATMENT APPROACHES

Pharmacological Management

Pharmacological management forms a cornerstone of treatment for colitis, aiming to alleviate symptoms, induce remission, and maintain long-term disease control. Various classes of medications are utilized in the management of colitis, targeting different aspects of the inflammatory process and immune dysregulation. In this section, we explore the pharmacological options available for the treatment of colitis, including aminosalicylates, corticosteroids, immunomodulators, biologic therapies, and antibiotics.

Aminosalicylates

Aminosalicylates, also known as 5-aminosalicylic acid (5-ASA) derivatives, are first-line agents for inducing and maintaining remission in mild to moderate colitis. These medications exert anti-inflammatory effects by inhibiting prostaglandin synthesis, scavenging free radicals, and modulating immune responses within the intestinal mucosa. Commonly used aminosalicylates include:

- **Mesalamine:** Mesalamine is the mainstay of aminosalicylate therapy, available in various formulations including oral tablets, capsules, enemas, and suppositories. Mesalamine acts topically within the colon, delivering anti-inflammatory effects directly to the inflamed mucosa. It is effective for inducing and maintaining remission in ulcerative colitis, with minimal systemic side effects.
- **Sulfasalazine:** Sulfasalazine consists of mesalamine linked to sulfapyridine by an azo bond, requiring colonic bacteria to cleave and release the active moiety. It is effective for both induction and maintenance of remission in ulcerative colitis, although its use may be limited by adverse effects such as headache, nausea, and reversible oligospermia in males.
- **Olsalazine:** Olsalazine is a dimer of mesalamine molecules linked by an azo bond, similar to sulfasalazine but without the sulfapyridine component. Olsalazine undergoes colonic cleavage to release mesalamine, providing targeted anti-inflammatory therapy to the affected mucosa. It is effective for mild to moderate ulcerative colitis, with a lower risk of adverse effects compared to sulfasalazine.

Corticosteroids

Corticosteroids are potent anti-inflammatory agents used for the induction of remission in moderate to severe colitis, particularly in cases refractory to aminosalicylates. These medications exert immunosuppressive effects by inhibiting cytokine production, reducing leukocyte migration, and suppressing inflammatory signaling pathways. Commonly used corticosteroids include:

- **Prednisone:** Prednisone is the oral corticosteroid of choice for the induction of remission in moderate to severe colitis. It is rapidly absorbed and metabolized in the liver to its active form, prednisolone, exerting systemic anti-inflammatory effects throughout the body. Prednisone is effective for short-term management of colitis flares but is associated with significant adverse effects with long-term use.

- **Budesonide:** Budesonide is a second-generation corticosteroid with high topical potency and low systemic bioavailability due to extensive first-pass metabolism in the liver. It is available in oral and rectal formulations for the treatment of mild to moderate colitis, offering localized anti-inflammatory therapy with reduced risk of systemic side effects compared to prednisone.

Immunomodulators

Immunomodulators are steroid-sparing agents used for the maintenance of remission in colitis and for the management of corticosteroid-dependent or refractory disease. These medications exert immunosuppressive effects by inhibiting T cell activation, modulating cytokine production, and promoting immune tolerance. Commonly used immunomodulators include:

- **Azathioprine:** Azathioprine is a purine analogue that suppresses T cell proliferation and inhibits DNA synthesis, leading to immunosuppression. It is effective for maintaining remission and reducing corticosteroid requirements in colitis patients, although its onset of action may be delayed, requiring several weeks to achieve therapeutic effect.
- **6-Mercaptopurine (6-MP):** 6-Mercaptopurine is a metabolite of azathioprine with similar immunosuppressive properties, acting as a purine antagonist to inhibit DNA and RNA synthesis in

proliferating cells. It is used as an alternative to azathioprine for maintenance therapy in colitis patients, particularly in cases intolerant or resistant to azathioprine therapy.

Biologic Therapies

Biologic therapies represent a major advancement in the treatment of colitis, targeting specific cytokines or immune pathways implicated in disease pathogenesis. These medications are reserved for patients with moderate to severe colitis refractory to conventional therapies or corticosteroid-dependent disease. Commonly used biologic therapies include:

- **Anti-Tumor Necrosis Factor (TNF) Agents:** Anti-TNF agents, such as infliximab, adalimumab, and golimumab, target the pro-inflammatory cytokine TNF-α to suppress immune responses and reduce mucosal inflammation in colitis. They are effective for inducing and maintaining remission in moderate to severe colitis, either as monotherapy or in combination with immunomodulators.
- **Anti-Integrin Antibodies:** Anti-integrin antibodies, such as vedolizumab and integrilin, target integrin molecules involved in leukocyte trafficking and adhesion to the intestinal mucosa. They selectively inhibit gut-specific lymphocyte homing and activation, offering targeted therapy for mucosal inflammation in colitis patients refractory to conventional treatments.

Antibiotics

Antibiotics are occasionally used in the management of colitis, particularly in cases where bacterial overgrowth, infection, or dysbiosis contribute to disease pathogenesis. While not typically considered first-line therapy for ulcerative colitis or

Crohn's disease, antibiotics may have a role in certain clinical scenarios, including:

- **Infectious Colitis:** Antibiotics are essential for the treatment of infectious colitis caused by bacterial, viral, or parasitic pathogens. In cases of bacterial colitis, such as Clostridioides difficile infection or bacterial overgrowth, antibiotics targeting the specific pathogen are prescribed to eradicate the infection and alleviate symptoms. Commonly used antibiotics for infectious colitis include metronidazole, vancomycin, fluoroquinolones, and rifaximin.
- **Perianal Fistulas:** Antibiotics may be used adjunctively in the management of perianal fistulas associated with Crohn's disease. They help control secondary infections, reduce perianal inflammation, and promote wound healing in fistula tracts. Antibiotics with anaerobic coverage, such as metronidazole and ciprofloxacin, are often prescribed in combination with immunomodulators or biologic therapies for perianal fistula management.
- **Postoperative Prophylaxis:** Antibiotics may be administered prophylactically perioperatively to reduce the risk of surgical site infections and postoperative complications in colitis patients undergoing gastrointestinal surgery. Prophylactic antibiotics are prescribed based on surgical factors, patient characteristics, and the presence of risk factors for surgical site infections. Commonly used antibiotics for postoperative prophylaxis include cephalosporins, metronidazole, and fluoroquinolones.

Considerations and Limitations:

While antibiotics may offer benefits in certain clinical contexts, their use in colitis management is not without considerations and limitations:

- **Risk of Microbiome Disruption:** Antibiotic therapy can disrupt the gut microbiota, altering microbial diversity, composition, and function. Prolonged or indiscriminate use of antibiotics may lead to dysbiosis, antibiotic resistance, and secondary infections, exacerbating mucosal inflammation and compromising host-microbiome interactions in colitis.
- **Selective Antibiotic Use:** Antibiotics should be prescribed judiciously and selectively in colitis management, targeting specific indications such as infectious colitis, perianal fistulas, or postoperative prophylaxis. Empirical antibiotic therapy without confirmed indications or appropriate diagnostic evaluation may lead to unnecessary antibiotic exposure, adverse effects, and treatment failures in colitis patients.
- **Combination Therapy:** Antibiotics are often used in combination with other pharmacological agents, such as aminosalicylates, corticosteroids, immunomodulators, or biologic therapies, for optimal management of colitis. Combination therapy may enhance treatment efficacy, reduce inflammation, and prevent disease relapse in colitis patients with complex or refractory disease phenotypes.

Future Directions:

Future research efforts are needed to elucidate the role of antibiotics in colitis management, exploring their impact on microbial communities, immune responses, and disease outcomes. Key areas for future investigation include:

- **Microbiome Modulation:** Advancements in microbiome research may identify novel targets for antibiotic therapy, enabling targeted modulation of microbial communities to restore microbial homeostasis, enhance

mucosal healing, and improve clinical outcomes in colitis patients.
- **Precision Antibiotic Therapy:** Integration of microbial profiling, host genetics, and clinical phenotyping may enable precision antibiotic therapy in colitis management, tailoring antibiotic regimens to individual patient characteristics, disease subtypes, and microbial signatures for optimized treatment efficacy and safety.
- **Antibiotic Stewardship:** Implementation of antibiotic stewardship programs and guidelines is essential to promote rational antibiotic use, minimize antimicrobial resistance, and preserve the effectiveness of antibiotics in colitis management. Multidisciplinary collaboration between gastroenterologists, infectious disease specialists, and antimicrobial stewardship teams is critical for promoting judicious antibiotic prescribing practices and optimizing patient care in colitis.

In conclusion, while antibiotics play a limited role in the management of colitis, they are valuable therapeutic agents in specific clinical scenarios such as infectious colitis, perianal fistulas, and postoperative prophylaxis. Considerations regarding antibiotic selection, timing, and duration are important to minimize adverse effects, preserve microbiome integrity, and optimize treatment outcomes in colitis patients. Future research endeavors will further elucidate the role of antibiotics in colitis management, exploring innovative strategies for microbiome modulation, precision antibiotic therapy, and antibiotic stewardship to improve patient care and outcomes.

Surgical Interventions

Surgical interventions play a crucial role in the management of colitis, particularly in cases of severe disease refractory to medical therapy, complications such as strictures or fistulas, or when malignancy is suspected. Surgical procedures aim to alleviate symptoms, remove diseased tissue, and improve quality of life in colitis patients. In this section, we explore the common surgical interventions utilized in the management of colitis, including colectomy with ileal pouch-anal anastomosis, strictureplasty, and resection of diseased bowel segments.

Colectomy and Ileal Pouch-Anal Anastomosis (IPAA)

Colectomy with ileal pouch-anal anastomosis (IPAA), also known as restorative proctocolectomy, is a surgical procedure performed primarily for the treatment of ulcerative colitis and familial adenomatous polyposis (FAP). The procedure involves removal of the entire colon and rectum, followed by creation of a pouch from the terminal ileum and anastomosis to the anus, allowing for preservation of bowel continuity and restoration of fecal continence. Key aspects of colectomy with IPAA include:

- **Indications:** Colectomy with IPAA is indicated for patients with refractory ulcerative colitis unresponsive to medical therapy, those with dysplasia or malignancy, or those with severe complications such as toxic megacolon, colonic perforation, or fulminant colitis. It is also performed in patients with FAP to prevent colorectal cancer development.
- **Surgical Technique:** The surgical procedure involves a staged approach, with initial subtotal colectomy followed by creation of the ileal pouch and anastomosis to the anus. The pouch is typically constructed in a J-shaped or S-shaped configuration from the distal ileum, preserving adequate length and capacity for fecal storage. The pouch is then anastomosed to the anal canal, restoring intestinal continuity and preserving anal sphincter function.

- **Outcomes:** Colectomy with IPAA offers durable symptomatic relief and excellent functional outcomes in the majority of patients with ulcerative colitis. It eliminates colonic inflammation, reduces disease recurrence, and eliminates the risk of colorectal cancer in patients with FAP. However, it is associated with potential complications such as pouchitis, anastomotic leakage, pelvic sepsis, and pouch dysfunction, which may necessitate revision surgery or pouch removal in some cases.

Strictureplasty

Strictureplasty is a surgical procedure performed to alleviate intestinal strictures and obstructive symptoms in patients with Crohn's disease. Unlike resection, which involves removal of diseased bowel segments, strictureplasty preserves bowel length and avoids the need for permanent ostomy formation. Key aspects of strictureplasty include:

- **Indications:** Strictureplasty is indicated for patients with Crohn's disease complicated by fibrostenotic strictures causing obstructive symptoms, such as abdominal pain, nausea, vomiting, or bowel obstruction. It is particularly useful in cases where multiple strictures or extensive bowel involvement preclude extensive resection.
- **Surgical Technique:** The surgical procedure involves longitudinal incision and closure of strictured bowel segments to widen the intestinal lumen and relieve obstruction. Various strictureplasty techniques may be employed, including Heineke-Mikulicz, Finney, or Michelassi strictureplasty, depending on the location and length of the stricture. Strictureplasty may be performed laparoscopically or through open surgical approaches.
- **Outcomes:** Strictureplasty is associated with favorable

outcomes in selected patients with Crohn's disease, providing effective relief of obstructive symptoms and preserving bowel length. It avoids the need for extensive resection and permanent ostomy formation, maintaining intestinal continuity and functional integrity. However, it may be associated with risks of anastomotic leakage, stricture recurrence, and disease progression in some cases.

Resection of Diseased Bowel Segments

Resection of diseased bowel segments is a common surgical intervention performed in patients with colitis, particularly in cases of Crohn's disease or complicated ulcerative colitis. The procedure involves removal of diseased or inflamed bowel segments, followed by primary anastomosis or creation of a temporary or permanent ostomy, depending on disease severity and surgical considerations. Key aspects of bowel resection include:

- **Indications:** Resection of diseased bowel segments is indicated for patients with Crohn's disease complicated by strictures, fistulas, abscesses, or refractory medical therapy. It is also performed in cases of ulcerative colitis with severe inflammation, dysplasia, or malignancy unresponsive to medical management.
- **Surgical Technique:** The surgical procedure involves identification and isolation of diseased bowel segments, followed by careful dissection and mobilization of the affected bowel. Diseased segments are then resected with adequate margins of healthy tissue, and intestinal continuity is restored through primary anastomosis or creation of a temporary or permanent ostomy, depending on surgical considerations.
- **Outcomes:** Resection of diseased bowel segments provides symptomatic relief, disease control, and

potential for long-term remission in patients with colitis. It eliminates inflamed or obstructed bowel segments, reduces disease recurrence, and improves overall quality of life. However, it may be associated with risks of anastomotic leakage, postoperative complications, and disease recurrence in some cases.

In conclusion, surgical interventions play a vital role in the management of colitis, providing effective relief of symptoms, control of disease complications, and improvement in quality of life for patients with refractory or severe disease. Colectomy with ileal pouch-anal anastomosis, strictureplasty, and resection of diseased bowel segments are important surgical options utilized in the treatment of colitis, tailored to individual patient characteristics, disease phenotype, and surgical considerations. Collaborative decision-making between gastroenterologists, colorectal surgeons, and multidisciplinary care teams is essential for optimizing surgical outcomes and ensuring comprehensive care for colitis patients.

Nutritional Therapy

Nutritional therapy plays a significant role in the management of colitis, providing essential nutrients, modulating immune responses, and promoting mucosal healing. Various dietary interventions are utilized to alleviate symptoms, reduce inflammation, and optimize nutritional status in colitis patients. In this section, we explore the different nutritional strategies employed in the management of colitis, including enteral nutrition, elemental diets, and dietary modifications with supplements.

Enteral Nutrition

Enteral nutrition involves the delivery of liquid nutritional formulas directly into the gastrointestinal tract, providing essential nutrients while resting the inflamed bowel. It is commonly used as adjunctive therapy in the management of active colitis, particularly in pediatric patients or those with severe disease refractory to medical therapy. Key aspects of enteral nutrition include:

- **Mechanism of Action:** Enteral nutrition exerts anti-inflammatory effects by reducing mucosal exposure to dietary antigens, modulating gut microbiota composition, and promoting mucosal healing. It provides easily absorbable nutrients, vitamins, and minerals without the need for digestion, supporting metabolic requirements and immune function.
- **Indications:** Enteral nutrition is indicated for patients with active colitis, particularly those with pediatric-onset disease, growth failure, or severe inflammation unresponsive to conventional medical therapy. It may be used as primary therapy in selected cases or as adjunctive therapy alongside pharmacological interventions to induce remission and optimize nutritional status.
- **Formulations:** Enteral nutrition formulas are available in various compositions, including polymeric, semi-elemental, or elemental formulations, depending on patient age, disease severity, and nutritional requirements. Polymeric formulas contain intact proteins, carbohydrates, and fats, suitable for most patients with intact gastrointestinal function. Semi-elemental and elemental formulas contain partially or fully hydrolyzed nutrients, designed for patients with malabsorption or impaired digestion.
- **Delivery Methods:** Enteral nutrition may be delivered via nasogastric tube, nasojejunal tube, or gastrostomy tube, depending on patient preferences, nutritional requirements, and gastrointestinal function. Continuous

infusion or intermittent bolus feeding regimens may be used, tailored to individual patient tolerance, compliance, and nutritional goals.
- **Outcomes:** Enteral nutrition has been shown to be effective in inducing remission, reducing disease activity, and improving nutritional status in colitis patients, particularly in pediatric populations. It is associated with fewer adverse effects compared to corticosteroids, such as growth suppression, bone density loss, or metabolic disturbances. However, compliance with enteral nutrition regimens may be challenging, requiring close monitoring, nutritional support, and multidisciplinary care.

Elemental Diets

Elemental diets, also known as amino acid-based diets, consist of predigested nutrients in free amino acid or peptide form, designed to minimize antigenic stimulation and facilitate absorption in patients with severe malabsorption or intestinal inflammation. They are utilized in the management of active colitis, particularly in cases refractory to conventional therapies or those with extensive small bowel involvement. Key aspects of elemental diets include:

- **Mechanism of Action:** Elemental diets provide predigested nutrients that require minimal digestive processing, bypassing inflamed or damaged segments of the gastrointestinal tract. They reduce antigenic stimulation, bowel inflammation, and mucosal injury, promoting mucosal healing and restoration of barrier function.
- **Indications:** Elemental diets are indicated for patients with severe colitis, extensive small bowel involvement, malabsorption syndromes, or severe protein-calorie malnutrition. They may be used as primary therapy

to induce remission or as adjunctive therapy alongside pharmacological interventions in cases refractory to conventional treatments.

- **Formulations:** Elemental diets are available as ready-to-use liquid formulas containing free amino acids, peptides, carbohydrates, fats, vitamins, and minerals in predigested forms. They are hypoallergenic, gluten-free, and lactose-free, suitable for patients with food allergies, intolerances, or inflammatory bowel disease.
- **Delivery Methods:** Elemental diets may be administered orally, via enteral feeding tubes, or parenterally, depending on patient preferences, nutritional requirements, and gastrointestinal function. Continuous infusion or intermittent bolus feeding regimens may be used, tailored to individual patient tolerance, compliance, and nutritional goals.
- **Outcomes:** Elemental diets have been shown to be effective in inducing remission, reducing disease activity, and improving nutritional status in patients with severe colitis or malabsorption syndromes. They are associated with minimal antigenic stimulation, reduced inflammation, and enhanced mucosal healing compared to conventional diets or total parenteral nutrition. However, compliance with elemental diets may be challenging due to taste, palatability, and cost considerations.

Dietary Modifications and Supplements

Dietary modifications and supplements play a complementary role in the management of colitis, providing symptom relief, reducing inflammation, and optimizing nutritional status. Various dietary approaches and nutritional supplements are utilized to alleviate symptoms, modulate immune responses, and support mucosal healing in colitis patients. Key aspects of dietary modifications and supplements include:

- **Anti-Inflammatory Diet:** Anti-inflammatory diets, such as the Mediterranean diet, low FODMAP diet, or specific carbohydrate diet (SCD), focus on reducing dietary triggers of inflammation, such as refined carbohydrates, processed foods, and pro-inflammatory fats, while emphasizing whole grains, fruits, vegetables, lean proteins, and healthy fats. These diets may help alleviate symptoms, improve gut microbiota composition, and reduce disease activity in colitis patients.
- **Dietary Fiber Supplementation:** Soluble fiber supplements, such as psyllium husk, methylcellulose, or acacia fiber, may help alleviate symptoms of constipation, diarrhea, or abdominal discomfort in colitis patients. They provide bulking effects, stool normalization, and prebiotic properties, promoting microbial diversity, fermentation, and short-chain fatty acid production in the colon.
- **Omega-3 Fatty Acids:** Omega-3 fatty acids, found in fatty fish, flaxseeds, chia seeds, and walnuts, have anti-inflammatory properties and may help reduce mucosal inflammation, cytokine production, and disease activity in colitis patients. Omega-3 fatty acid supplementation, either through dietary sources or fish oil supplements, may provide symptomatic relief and support mucosal healing in colitis management.
- **Probiotics and Prebiotics:** Probiotics are live microorganisms that confer health benefits when consumed in adequate amounts, while prebiotics are non-digestible carbohydrates that selectively stimulate the growth and activity of beneficial gut microbiota. Probiotics and prebiotics may help restore gut microbial balance, enhance mucosal barrier function, and modulate immune responses in colitis patients, promoting gut health and reducing disease severity.
- **Vitamin and Mineral Supplements:** Vitamin and

mineral deficiencies are common in colitis patients due to malabsorption, dietary restrictions, or disease-related inflammation. Supplementation with vitamins (such as vitamin D, vitamin B12, folate) and minerals (such as iron, calcium, zinc) may help correct nutritional deficiencies, support immune function, and promote mucosal healing in colitis management.

In conclusion, nutritional therapy plays an integral role in the management of colitis, providing essential nutrients, modulating immune responses, and promoting mucosal healing. Enteral nutrition, elemental diets, dietary modifications, and nutritional supplements are important adjunctive strategies utilized to alleviate symptoms, reduce inflammation, and optimize nutritional status in colitis patients. Individualized dietary plans should be tailored to the patient's specific needs, disease phenotype, nutritional status, and treatment goals, with close monitoring and collaboration between gastroenterologists, registered dietitians, and other members of the healthcare team. While nutritional therapy alone may not be sufficient to achieve remission in all cases of colitis, it plays a crucial role in comprehensive disease management, complementing pharmacological interventions, surgical treatments, and lifestyle modifications to improve patient outcomes and quality of life.

Parenteral Nutrition

Parenteral nutrition, also known as total parenteral nutrition (TPN), is a form of nutritional support delivered intravenously to patients unable to tolerate oral or enteral feeding due to severe colitis, bowel obstruction, or malabsorption. It provides essential nutrients, vitamins, minerals, and calories directly into the bloodstream, bypassing the gastrointestinal tract. Parenteral nutrition is reserved for patients with severe malnutrition, intestinal failure, or contraindications to enteral nutrition. Key aspects of parenteral nutrition include:

- **Indications:** Parenteral nutrition is indicated for patients with severe colitis or complications such as bowel obstruction, fistulas, or extensive small bowel involvement, rendering enteral feeding impractical or ineffective. It may be used as temporary or long-term therapy to provide adequate nutritional support and prevent further deterioration of nutritional status in critically ill patients.
- **Composition:** Parenteral nutrition solutions are customized to meet individual patient requirements, comprising dextrose, amino acids, lipids, electrolytes, vitamins, and trace elements in predetermined concentrations. The composition of parenteral nutrition is adjusted based on patient's energy expenditure, protein requirements, fluid balance, and metabolic needs, with close monitoring of biochemical parameters and nutritional status.
- **Delivery Methods:** Parenteral nutrition is administered through a central venous catheter, such as a central line or peripherally inserted central catheter (PICC), to ensure adequate venous access and delivery of nutrition directly into the central circulation. The infusion rate, duration, and composition of parenteral nutrition are carefully titrated based on patient tolerance, metabolic demands, and clinical response, with regular monitoring of electrolytes, glucose levels, and liver function tests.
- **Outcomes:** Parenteral nutrition provides essential nutritional support and prevents malnutrition-related complications in patients unable to tolerate oral or enteral feeding due to severe colitis or gastrointestinal dysfunction. It maintains adequate caloric intake, prevents muscle wasting, and supports immune function in critically ill patients, improving overall nutritional status and clinical outcomes. However, parenteral nutrition is associated with risks of

catheter-related infections, metabolic complications, and liver dysfunction, requiring close monitoring and multidisciplinary management.

In conclusion, parenteral nutrition plays a crucial role in the management of severe colitis, providing essential nutrients, calories, and fluids to patients unable to tolerate oral or enteral feeding due to gastrointestinal dysfunction. It offers a lifeline for critically ill patients with severe malnutrition, bowel obstruction, or complications of colitis, ensuring adequate nutritional support and preventing further deterioration of nutritional status. However, parenteral nutrition should be used judiciously, considering the risks and benefits, and tailored to individual patient needs, with close monitoring and interdisciplinary collaboration to optimize patient outcomes and quality of life.

Complementary and Alternative Medicine

Complementary and alternative medicine (CAM) encompasses a diverse range of therapeutic approaches and practices used alongside conventional medical treatments to manage colitis. These interventions may offer additional benefits in symptom relief, immune modulation, and overall well-being for colitis patients. In this section, we explore various CAM modalities, including probiotics and prebiotics, herbal remedies, and mind-body practices.

Probiotics and Prebiotics

Probiotics are live microorganisms that confer health benefits when consumed in adequate amounts, while prebiotics are non-digestible carbohydrates that selectively stimulate the growth and activity of beneficial gut microbiota. Both probiotics and prebiotics play a crucial role in modulating gut microbiota composition, enhancing mucosal barrier function, and regulating immune responses in colitis patients. Key aspects of probiotics and prebiotics include:

- **Mechanism of Action:** Probiotics exert beneficial effects by colonizing the gastrointestinal tract, competing with pathogenic bacteria for nutrients and adhesion sites, and producing antimicrobial substances such as short-chain fatty acids (SCFAs) and bacteriocins. Prebiotics serve as substrates for beneficial gut bacteria, promoting their growth and activity while inhibiting the proliferation of pathogenic organisms.
- **Indications:** Probiotics and prebiotics are indicated for patients with colitis, particularly those with inflammatory bowel disease (IBD), including ulcerative colitis and Crohn's disease. They may help alleviate symptoms such as abdominal pain, bloating, diarrhea, and inflammation, while promoting gut health, microbial diversity, and immune regulation.
- **Strains and Formulations:** Probiotics are available in various strains and formulations, including Lactobacillus, Bifidobacterium, and Saccharomyces species, each with unique properties and mechanisms of action. Prebiotics include oligosaccharides, such as fructooligosaccharides (FOS) and galactooligosaccharides (GOS), as well as dietary fibers such as inulin, resistant starch, and soluble fibers.
- **Clinical Evidence:** Clinical studies have demonstrated mixed results regarding the efficacy of probiotics and prebiotics in colitis management. While some trials have shown beneficial effects on disease activity, symptom improvement, and mucosal healing, others have reported no significant differences compared to placebo. The effectiveness of probiotics and prebiotics may vary depending on factors such as strain selection, dosage,

duration of treatment, and patient characteristics.

Herbal Remedies

Herbal remedies, derived from plant sources, have been used for centuries in traditional medicine systems to alleviate gastrointestinal symptoms, reduce inflammation, and promote healing in colitis patients. While scientific evidence supporting the efficacy of herbal remedies in colitis management is limited, some herbs may possess anti-inflammatory, antioxidant, and immunomodulatory properties. Key aspects of herbal remedies include:

- **Commonly Used Herbs:** Several herbs have been studied for their potential therapeutic effects in colitis, including aloe vera, turmeric (curcumin), Boswellia serrata (frankincense), slippery elm, chamomile, and licorice root. These herbs may exert anti-inflammatory effects, modulate immune responses, and promote mucosal healing through various mechanisms of action.
- **Mechanisms of Action:** Herbal remedies may modulate inflammatory pathways, such as NF-κB signaling, cytokine production, and leukocyte migration, leading to reduced mucosal inflammation and tissue damage. They may also scavenge free radicals, inhibit prostaglandin synthesis, and enhance tissue repair mechanisms in the gastrointestinal tract.
- **Formulations and Dosages:** Herbal remedies are available in various formulations, including teas, tinctures, capsules, and extracts, each with different concentrations and bioavailability. Dosages may vary depending on the herb, its preparation, and the severity of colitis symptoms. It is essential to consult with a healthcare provider or qualified herbalist before using herbal remedies, as they may interact with medications or exacerbate underlying health conditions.

- **Safety and Efficacy:** While herbal remedies are generally considered safe when used appropriately, they may have potential side effects, interactions, or contraindications, particularly in patients with colitis or other medical conditions. It is essential to use caution and follow evidence-based guidelines when incorporating herbal remedies into colitis management, seeking guidance from healthcare professionals to ensure safety and efficacy.

Mind-Body Practices

Mind-body practices encompass a variety of techniques and interventions aimed at promoting mental, emotional, and physical well-being through the integration of mind and body. These practices may help reduce stress, anxiety, and depression, which are common comorbidities in colitis patients, while enhancing coping mechanisms and resilience. Key aspects of mind-body practices include:

- **Stress Reduction Techniques:** Mindfulness meditation, guided imagery, progressive muscle relaxation, and deep breathing exercises are examples of stress reduction techniques that may benefit colitis patients. These practices help induce a state of relaxation, reduce sympathetic nervous system activity, and promote parasympathetic activation, leading to reduced inflammation and improved gut function.
- **Yoga and Tai Chi:** Yoga and Tai Chi are mind-body practices that combine physical postures, breathing techniques, and meditation to promote balance, flexibility, and relaxation. They may help alleviate gastrointestinal symptoms, improve bowel function, and enhance quality of life in colitis patients by reducing stress, improving body awareness, and fostering mind-body integration.

- **Biofeedback and Hypnotherapy:** Biofeedback and hypnotherapy are therapeutic techniques that enable individuals to gain conscious control over physiological processes, such as heart rate, blood pressure, and muscle tension, through feedback and mental imagery. These modalities may help colitis patients manage symptoms such as abdominal pain, bloating, and urgency by promoting relaxation, reducing visceral hypersensitivity, and modulating autonomic nervous system function.
- **Cognitive-Behavioral Therapy (CBT):** CBT is a psychotherapeutic approach that focuses on identifying and modifying maladaptive thought patterns and behaviors associated with stress, anxiety, and depression. It helps colitis patients develop coping strategies, problem-solving skills, and resilience to better manage the emotional and psychological challenges of living with a chronic illness. CBT may improve mood, quality of life, and treatment adherence in colitis patients, reducing the impact of psychological factors on disease outcomes.
- **Supportive Counseling and Group Therapy:** Supportive counseling and group therapy provide opportunities for colitis patients to express emotions, share experiences, and receive emotional support from peers and mental health professionals. These interventions foster a sense of belonging, validation, and understanding, reducing feelings of isolation and stigma associated with colitis. They promote social connectedness, coping skills, and self-empowerment in navigating the challenges of living with a chronic illness.
- **Dietary and Lifestyle Counseling:** Dietary and lifestyle counseling is an integral component of mind-body practices in colitis management, emphasizing the importance of healthy eating habits, regular physical activity, adequate sleep, and stress management techniques. Healthcare providers and registered

dietitians collaborate with colitis patients to develop personalized nutrition plans, exercise routines, and self-care strategies tailored to individual needs and preferences. These interventions promote holistic well-being, optimize disease management, and enhance quality of life in colitis patients.

In conclusion, mind-body practices offer valuable adjunctive therapies in the management of colitis, addressing the interconnectedness of mental, emotional, and physical health in disease outcomes. Probiotics and prebiotics may modulate gut microbiota composition and immune function, herbal remedies may exert anti-inflammatory and antioxidant effects, and mind-body practices may reduce stress, anxiety, and depression. Integrating these CAM modalities with conventional medical treatments, surgical interventions, and lifestyle modifications provides a comprehensive approach to colitis management, promoting holistic well-being and improving patient outcomes. Collaborative decision-making between healthcare providers, patients, and CAM practitioners is essential to ensure safe, effective, and patient-centered care in colitis management.

CHAPTER 7: COMPLICATIONS AND PROGNOSIS

Colonic Complications

Colonic complications are significant concerns in the management of colitis, potentially leading to severe morbidity and impacting the overall prognosis of affected individuals. These complications arise from the chronic inflammation and structural changes within the colon, manifesting with a diverse range of clinical presentations and requiring prompt recognition and intervention. In this section, we explore the common colonic complications associated with various forms of colitis, including ulcerative colitis, Crohn's disease, and other inflammatory conditions.

Toxic Megacolon

Toxic megacolon is a life-threatening complication characterized by severe colonic dilation (>6 cm) and systemic toxicity, often associated with fulminant colitis or severe inflammation involving the entire colon. It presents with abdominal distension, severe pain, fever, tachycardia, and signs of systemic inflammation, such as leukocytosis and elevated inflammatory markers. Complications of toxic megacolon include colonic perforation, sepsis, and multiorgan failure, requiring urgent medical intervention, intravenous corticosteroids, bowel rest, and close monitoring in a specialized care setting.

Colonic Perforation

Colonic perforation is a serious complication characterized by the breach of the colonic wall, leading to the leakage of intestinal contents into the peritoneal cavity and causing peritonitis, sepsis, and systemic inflammation. It may occur secondary to severe inflammation, ischemia, or mechanical obstruction, particularly in patients with ulcerative colitis, Crohn's disease, or ischemic colitis. Clinical features of colonic perforation include sudden onset of severe abdominal pain, guarding, rebound tenderness, and signs of systemic toxicity, necessitating emergent surgical evaluation, exploration, and repair.

Colonic Strictures

Colonic strictures are fibrotic narrowing of the colonic lumen, resulting from chronic inflammation, scarring, and tissue remodeling in response to repeated injury or healing processes. They may occur in patients with Crohn's disease, ulcerative colitis, or radiation colitis, leading to obstructive symptoms, such as abdominal pain, bloating, constipation, or diarrhea. Complications of colonic strictures include bowel obstruction, perforation, and fistula formation, requiring endoscopic evaluation, balloon dilation, or surgical intervention to alleviate symptoms and restore luminal patency.

Fistulas and Abscesses

Fistulas and abscesses are abnormal communications or collections of pus within or around the colon, resulting from chronic inflammation, tissue necrosis, and bacterial overgrowth. They may occur in patients with Crohn's disease, diverticulitis, or infectious colitis, presenting with symptoms such as fever, abdominal pain, rectal discharge, or perirectal swelling. Complications of fistulas and abscesses include sepsis, peritonitis, and systemic infection, requiring drainage, antibiotics, and surgical intervention to prevent further complications and promote healing.

Colorectal Cancer

Colorectal cancer is a long-term complication of colitis, particularly in patients with longstanding ulcerative colitis or Crohn's colitis involving the colon. Chronic inflammation, mucosal injury, and dysregulated immune responses contribute to the development of dysplasia and malignant transformation over time. Surveillance colonoscopy with targeted biopsies is recommended in colitis patients to detect early neoplastic changes, such as dysplasia or carcinoma, and initiate appropriate management, including surgical resection, endoscopic mucosal resection, or chemoprevention strategies.

In conclusion, colonic complications are significant considerations in the management of colitis, potentially leading to severe morbidity and mortality if not promptly recognized and treated. Toxic megacolon, colonic perforation, strictures, fistulas, abscesses, and colorectal cancer are among the common complications encountered in patients with colitis, requiring a multidisciplinary approach involving gastroenterologists, colorectal surgeons, radiologists, and pathologists. Early recognition, appropriate intervention, and close monitoring are essential to optimize outcomes and prevent long-term sequelae in affected individuals.

Extraintestinal Manifestations

Extraintestinal manifestations (EIMs) are a diverse group of clinical conditions that can occur in patients with colitis, affecting organs and systems outside the gastrointestinal tract. These manifestations often arise from the systemic inflammatory nature of colitis, autoimmune processes, or shared genetic predispositions. Recognizing and managing EIMs are crucial aspects of comprehensive colitis care, as they can significantly impact patient outcomes and quality of life. In this section, we explore the common extraintestinal manifestations associated with colitis, including ulcerative colitis, Crohn's disease, and other inflammatory bowel diseases.

Arthritis and Musculoskeletal Disorders

Arthritis and musculoskeletal disorders are among the most common extraintestinal manifestations of colitis, affecting up to one-third of patients with inflammatory bowel disease (IBD). These conditions encompass a spectrum of rheumatologic disorders, including peripheral arthritis, axial spondyloarthritis, sacroiliitis, and ankylosing spondylitis. Patients may present with joint pain, stiffness, swelling, and reduced range of motion, impacting mobility and functional status. Management of arthritis and musculoskeletal disorders in colitis patients may involve nonsteroidal anti-inflammatory drugs (NSAIDs), disease-modifying antirheumatic drugs (DMARDs), biologic therapies, physical therapy, and lifestyle modifications.

Dermatologic Manifestations

Dermatologic manifestations are common extraintestinal complications of colitis, affecting the skin, hair, and nails in various forms. These conditions include erythema nodosum, pyoderma gangrenosum, psoriasis, aphthous stomatitis, and perianal skin tags. Patients may present with painful nodules, ulcers, plaques, or vesicles, often correlating with disease activity or exacerbations of colitis. Dermatologic manifestations may require topical treatments, systemic medications, biologic therapies, or surgical interventions to alleviate symptoms and prevent complications.

Ocular Manifestations

Ocular manifestations are recognized extraintestinal complications of colitis, affecting the eyes and surrounding structures in a subset of patients. These conditions include episcleritis, scleritis, uveitis, and keratopathy, presenting with symptoms such as eye pain, redness, photophobia, and blurred vision. Ocular involvement may occur concurrently with colitis flares or independently, necessitating ophthalmologic evaluation, topical or systemic corticosteroids, immunosuppressive agents, and supportive measures to manage inflammation and preserve visual function.

Hepatobiliary Manifestations

Hepatobiliary manifestations are important extraintestinal complications of colitis, affecting the liver, gallbladder, and bile ducts in some patients. These conditions include primary sclerosing cholangitis (PSC), autoimmune hepatitis, cholelithiasis, and fatty liver disease. Patients may present with abnormal liver function tests, jaundice, pruritus, or hepatomegaly, indicating underlying hepatobiliary pathology. Management of hepatobiliary manifestations may involve immunosuppressive therapies, ursodeoxycholic acid (UDCA), cholecystectomy, liver transplantation, and lifestyle modifications to mitigate disease progression and complications.

Renal and Urologic Manifestations

Renal and urologic manifestations are recognized extraintestinal complications of colitis, affecting the kidneys, urinary tract, and associated structures in some patients. These conditions include nephrolithiasis, urinary tract infections (UTIs), interstitial nephritis, and amyloidosis. Patients may present with hematuria, flank pain, dysuria, or urinary urgency, reflecting underlying renal or urologic pathology. Management of renal and urologic manifestations may involve hydration, analgesia, antibiotics, immunosuppressive therapies, and surgical interventions to alleviate symptoms and prevent complications.

In conclusion, extraintestinal manifestations are common and diverse complications of colitis, affecting various organ systems outside the gastrointestinal tract. Arthritis, dermatologic conditions, ocular manifestations, hepatobiliary disorders, and renal/urologic complications are among the recognized EIMs encountered in patients with colitis, necessitating a multidisciplinary approach involving gastroenterologists, rheumatologists, dermatologists, ophthalmologists, hepatologists, nephrologists, and urologists. Early recognition, appropriate intervention, and close monitoring of EIMs are essential to optimize patient outcomes, minimize disease burden, and improve quality of life in individuals with colitis.

Risk of Colorectal Cancer

Colorectal cancer (CRC) represents a significant long-term complication of colitis, particularly in patients with longstanding and extensive disease involvement. Chronic inflammation, mucosal injury, and dysregulated immune responses contribute to the increased risk of CRC development in individuals with colitis, including ulcerative colitis (UC), Crohn's colitis, and other forms of inflammatory bowel disease (IBD). Understanding and managing the risk of CRC in colitis patients are essential aspects of disease monitoring and surveillance. In this section, we explore the factors contributing to the elevated risk of CRC in colitis and strategies for CRC screening, prevention, and management.

Factors Contributing to Increased CRC Risk

Several factors contribute to the heightened risk of CRC in patients with colitis:

- **Duration and Extent of Colitis:** The duration and extent of colitis are key determinants of CRC risk, with longer disease duration and extensive colonic involvement associated with higher malignancy rates. Patients with pancolitis (involving the entire colon) have a substantially increased risk of CRC compared to those with limited colitis involvement.
- **Severity of Inflammation:** The severity and intensity of colonic inflammation correlate with the risk of CRC development. Persistent and severe inflammation, characterized by frequent flares, mucosal ulceration, and crypt distortion, is associated with an elevated risk of dysplasia and malignant transformation over time.
- **Presence of Dysplasia:** The presence of dysplasia, characterized by abnormal cellular changes in the colonic epithelium, is a significant precursor to CRC development in colitis patients. Low-grade dysplasia confers a moderate risk of progression to CRC, while high-grade dysplasia is considered a more imminent threat requiring prompt intervention.
- **Family History of CRC:** A family history of CRC or related malignancies (such as Lynch syndrome) increases the risk of CRC in colitis patients. Genetic predispositions, inherited mutations, and shared environmental factors may contribute to the development of CRC in susceptible individuals.
- **Age at Diagnosis:** The age at colitis diagnosis influences the cumulative risk of CRC, with younger age at onset associated with a longer duration of disease exposure

and increased likelihood of malignancy over time.

CRC Screening and Surveillance

Given the heightened risk of CRC in colitis patients, regular screening and surveillance strategies are essential for early detection and intervention. Current guidelines recommend the following approaches for CRC screening and surveillance in colitis patients:

- **Colonoscopy:** Colonoscopy is the primary modality for CRC screening and surveillance in colitis patients, allowing direct visualization of the colonic mucosa, detection of dysplastic lesions, and targeted biopsies for histological evaluation. Patients with colitis should undergo surveillance colonoscopy at regular intervals, typically starting 8-10 years after diagnosis of extensive colitis or 15-20 years after diagnosis of left-sided colitis.
- **Interval of Surveillance:** The interval between surveillance colonoscopies depends on the presence and severity of colonic inflammation, the presence of dysplasia, and individual patient risk factors. Patients with no dysplasia or low-grade dysplasia may undergo surveillance colonoscopy every 1-3 years, while those with high-grade dysplasia may require more frequent monitoring or consideration for surgical intervention.
- **Chromoendoscopy and Advanced Imaging Techniques:** Chromoendoscopy, virtual chromoendoscopy (such as narrow-band imaging or blue light imaging), and other advanced imaging techniques may enhance the detection of dysplastic lesions and improve the accuracy of surveillance colonoscopy in colitis patients. These modalities may be considered in select cases, particularly for patients at high risk of CRC or those with suboptimal visualization of the colonic mucosa.

Chemoprevention Strategies

Chemoprevention strategies aim to reduce the risk of CRC development in colitis patients through the use of pharmacological agents with anti-inflammatory, immunomodulatory, or antineoplastic properties. Commonly studied chemopreventive agents include:

- **5-Aminosalicylates (5-ASAs):** 5-ASAs are anti-inflammatory medications commonly used in the management of colitis, which may also exert chemopreventive effects by reducing inflammation, inhibiting prostaglandin synthesis, and promoting mucosal healing. Long-term use of 5-ASAs has been associated with a reduced risk of CRC in colitis patients.
- **Immunomodulators:** Immunomodulatory agents, such as thiopurines (azathioprine, mercaptopurine) and methotrexate, may help reduce the risk of CRC in colitis patients by modulating immune responses, suppressing inflammation, and inhibiting cell proliferation. These medications may be considered in patients with refractory colitis or those at high risk of CRC.
- **Biologic Therapies:** Biologic therapies, including tumor necrosis factor (TNF) alpha inhibitors (e.g., infliximab, adalimumab), vedolizumab, and ustekinumab, target specific inflammatory pathways implicated in colitis pathogenesis and may have additional chemopreventive effects on CRC development. These medications are reserved for patients with moderate to severe colitis refractory to conventional therapies or those at high risk of CRC progression.
- **Aspirin and Nonsteroidal Anti-Inflammatory Drugs (NSAIDs):** Aspirin and NSAIDs have been investigated for their potential chemopreventive effects on CRC development in colitis patients. These medications may inhibit cyclooxygenase (COX) enzymes, reduce inflammation, and modulate cellular proliferation

pathways in the colonic mucosa. However, the use of aspirin and NSAIDs in colitis patients should be balanced against the risk of gastrointestinal bleeding and exacerbation of colonic inflammation.

Surgical Interventions

Surgical interventions may be necessary in colitis patients with advanced dysplasia, high-grade dysplasia, or CRC to remove the affected colonic segments and reduce the risk of disease progression. Surgical options for CRC risk reduction in colitis patients include:

- **Proctocolectomy with Ileal Pouch-Anal Anastomosis (IPAA):** Proctocolectomy with IPAA is a surgical procedure that involves the removal of the entire colon and rectum, followed by the creation of a reservoir (pouch) from the terminal ileum and anastomosis to the anal canal. This procedure preserves bowel continuity and eliminates the risk of CRC in colitis patients, offering a definitive treatment option for refractory disease or dysplasia.
- **Total Colectomy with End-Ileostomy:** Total colectomy with end-ileostomy is a surgical procedure that involves the removal of the entire colon and rectum, with diversion of the terminal ileum through an abdominal stoma (ileostomy). This procedure may be indicated in colitis patients with extensive colonic involvement, refractory inflammation, or complications such as toxic megacolon, perforation, or malignancy.
- **Surveillance after Surgical Resection:** Following surgical resection for CRC or dysplasia, colitis patients require continued surveillance to monitor for recurrence, metachronous lesions, or development of pouch-related complications. Surveillance colonoscopy, pouchoscopy, and imaging studies are performed at regular intervals to

detect early signs of disease recurrence or complications.

In conclusion, the risk of colorectal cancer (CRC) is a significant concern in patients with colitis, necessitating vigilant monitoring, surveillance, and intervention to mitigate disease progression and improve outcomes. Factors contributing to increased CRC risk in colitis patients include disease duration, severity of inflammation, presence of dysplasia, family history of CRC, and age at diagnosis. Screening and surveillance colonoscopy, chemoprevention strategies, surgical interventions, and multidisciplinary care are essential components of CRC risk management in colitis patients, aiming to optimize long-term outcomes and quality of life.

Factors Influencing Prognosis

The prognosis of colitis, including ulcerative colitis (UC), Crohn's disease, and other inflammatory bowel diseases (IBD), is influenced by various clinical, demographic, and pathological factors. Understanding these factors is crucial for predicting disease outcomes, guiding treatment decisions, and optimizing patient management. In this section, we explore the key factors influencing the prognosis of colitis and their implications for patient care.

Disease Severity and Extent

The severity and extent of colitis at the time of diagnosis are important prognostic indicators, with more extensive and severe disease associated with a higher risk of complications, disease progression, and adverse outcomes. Patients with pancolitis (involving the entire colon) or extensive colitis have an increased risk of colorectal cancer (CRC), toxic megacolon, hospitalization, and surgical intervention compared to those with limited colitis involvement. Disease severity is often assessed using clinical, endoscopic, and histological parameters, such as the Mayo score for UC or the Crohn's Disease Activity Index (CDAI) for Crohn's disease.

Complications and Extraintestinal Manifestations

The presence of complications, such as toxic megacolon, colonic perforation, strictures, fistulas, abscesses, or extraintestinal manifestations (EIMs), significantly impacts the prognosis of colitis. Complicated disease phenotypes are associated with a higher risk of hospitalization, surgical intervention, disability, and mortality, requiring aggressive management and close monitoring to prevent adverse outcomes. EIMs, including arthritis, dermatologic conditions, ocular manifestations, hepatobiliary disorders, and renal/urologic complications, may contribute to disease burden and impair quality of life in colitis patients, necessitating multidisciplinary care and targeted interventions.

Disease Course and Natural History

The disease course and natural history of colitis vary widely among patients, with some experiencing intermittent flares, remissions, and periods of stable disease, while others have chronic, progressive, or refractory disease requiring continuous medical therapy or surgical intervention. Factors influencing disease course and prognosis include age at diagnosis, disease duration, response to treatment, smoking status, genetic predispositions, and environmental triggers. Longitudinal studies and disease registries provide valuable insights into the natural history of colitis and predictors of disease outcomes over time.

Histopathological Features

Histopathological features observed on colonic biopsy specimens, such as degree of inflammation, presence of crypt distortion, depth of ulceration, presence of dysplasia, and degree of tissue fibrosis, provide important prognostic information regarding disease severity, progression, and response to treatment. Histological assessment is essential for confirming the diagnosis of colitis, characterizing disease activity, guiding treatment decisions, and monitoring disease progression over time. Histological remission, defined as resolution of inflammation and restoration of normal mucosal architecture, is a key therapeutic goal in colitis management and predicts favorable long-term outcomes.

Treatment Response and Adherence

The response to treatment and adherence to therapeutic regimens significantly influence the prognosis of colitis, with timely initiation of effective therapies associated with improved clinical outcomes, reduced disease activity, and enhanced quality of life. Patients who achieve and maintain remission with pharmacological, surgical, or adjunctive therapies have a lower risk of disease flares, hospitalization, and complications, while those with treatment resistance, intolerance, or nonadherence may experience disease progression, exacerbation of symptoms, and poorer prognosis over time. Tailored treatment approaches, patient education, shared decision-making, and multidisciplinary care are essential for optimizing treatment response and prognosis in colitis patients.

In conclusion, multiple factors influence the prognosis of colitis, including disease severity, extent, complications, extraintestinal manifestations, disease course, histopathological features, treatment response, and adherence. A comprehensive understanding of these factors is essential for risk stratification, prognostication, and personalized management of colitis patients, aiming to achieve optimal clinical outcomes, prevent complications, and improve quality of life. Multidisciplinary care, regular monitoring, and individualized treatment strategies are fundamental to optimizing prognosis and long-term outcomes in patients with colitis.

Quality of Life Considerations

Quality of life (QoL) considerations play a central role in the comprehensive management of colitis, encompassing physical, emotional, social, and functional aspects of well-being. Colitis, including ulcerative colitis (UC), Crohn's disease, and other inflammatory bowel diseases (IBD), can significantly impact various domains of patients' lives, affecting daily activities, relationships, work, leisure, and overall satisfaction. Understanding and addressing QoL issues are essential for optimizing patient care, enhancing treatment outcomes, and promoting holistic well-being. In this section, we explore the key QoL considerations in colitis management and strategies for improving QoL outcomes.

Symptom Management

Effective symptom management is paramount for improving QoL in colitis patients, as symptoms such as abdominal pain, diarrhea, rectal bleeding, fatigue, and urgency can significantly impair daily functioning and well-being. Tailored treatment approaches, including pharmacological therapies, dietary modifications, lifestyle interventions, and complementary therapies, aim to alleviate symptoms, reduce disease activity, and enhance patient comfort. Healthcare providers collaborate with patients to develop individualized symptom management plans, optimize treatment regimens, and minimize treatment-related side effects to improve QoL outcomes.

Psychological Support

Psychological support is essential for addressing the emotional and psychological impact of colitis on patients' mental health, coping strategies, and QoL. Living with a chronic illness such as colitis can lead to feelings of anxiety, depression, stress, isolation, and diminished self-esteem, highlighting the need for accessible and culturally sensitive mental health services. Cognitive-behavioral therapy (CBT), supportive counseling, mindfulness-based interventions, and peer support groups provide valuable resources for patients to cope with stress, manage emotions, enhance resilience, and improve QoL outcomes.

Social Support and Education

Social support and education play crucial roles in empowering colitis patients to actively participate in their care, make informed decisions, and advocate for their needs. Patient education programs, support networks, online forums, and patient advocacy organizations offer valuable opportunities for patients to connect with peers, access reliable information, share experiences, and learn self-management strategies. Peer mentors, patient navigators, and healthcare professionals serve as trusted sources of support, guidance, and encouragement in navigating the challenges of living with colitis and optimizing QoL outcomes.

Nutritional Counseling

Nutritional counseling is integral to addressing the dietary challenges and nutritional deficiencies commonly observed in colitis patients, optimizing dietary intake, and promoting gastrointestinal health. Registered dietitians collaborate with patients to develop personalized nutrition plans, identify trigger foods, manage food intolerances, and address malnutrition or weight loss associated with colitis flares or disease activity. Emphasizing a balanced diet, adequate hydration, supplementation as needed, and mindful eating practices can enhance nutritional status, symptom control, and QoL in colitis patients.

Physical Activity and Rehabilitation

Physical activity and rehabilitation interventions are important components of QoL management in colitis patients, promoting physical fitness, functional independence, and overall well-being. Regular exercise, tailored to individual preferences, capabilities, and disease activity, can improve cardiovascular health, muscle strength, flexibility, and fatigue levels, while reducing stress, anxiety, and depression associated with colitis. Physical therapists, occupational therapists, and exercise specialists collaborate with patients to develop personalized exercise programs, provide adaptive equipment, and address mobility limitations, fostering a sense of empowerment and self-efficacy in managing colitis-related symptoms and limitations.

Work and Vocational Support

Work and vocational support are essential for colitis patients to maintain employment, fulfill occupational roles, and achieve financial stability, despite the challenges posed by their illness. Flexible work arrangements, reasonable accommodations, and disability benefits may be necessary to accommodate colitis-related symptoms, medical appointments, and treatment regimens while ensuring job retention and productivity. Vocational rehabilitation programs, career counseling, and workplace accommodations facilitate the successful integration of colitis patients into the workforce, promoting financial independence, social inclusion, and QoL enhancement.

In conclusion, addressing QoL considerations is integral to optimizing the comprehensive management of colitis, enhancing patient well-being, and improving treatment outcomes. Symptom management, psychological support, social support, education, nutritional counseling, physical activity, rehabilitation, work/vocational support, and holistic care approaches are essential components of QoL-focused interventions in colitis management. Collaborative efforts among healthcare providers, patients, caregivers, and community resources are essential to address QoL challenges, promote resilience, and foster meaningful improvements in patients' lives.

CHAPTER 8: PREVENTIVE STRATEGIES

Lifestyle Modifications

Lifestyle modifications are integral components of the comprehensive management approach for colitis, including ulcerative colitis (UC), Crohn's disease, and other inflammatory bowel diseases (IBD). Adopting healthy lifestyle practices can help alleviate symptoms, reduce disease activity, improve quality of life, and complement medical therapies in the management of colitis. In this section, we explore various lifestyle modifications that may benefit individuals with colitis.

Dietary Modifications

Dietary modifications play a crucial role in managing symptoms and optimizing gastrointestinal health in colitis patients. While dietary triggers may vary among individuals, certain general principles can help guide dietary choices:

- **Low-Residue Diet:** A low-residue diet, emphasizing low-fiber foods that are easily digestible and less likely to irritate the gastrointestinal tract, may help reduce bowel movements, abdominal discomfort, and stool frequency

in colitis patients during flares.
- **Elimination of Trigger Foods:** Identifying and avoiding trigger foods that exacerbate symptoms, such as spicy foods, dairy products, caffeine, alcohol, and high-fat or high-fiber foods, can help minimize gastrointestinal distress and improve symptom control.
- **Probiotics and Prebiotics:** Incorporating probiotic-rich foods (e.g., yogurt, kefir, fermented vegetables) and prebiotic-containing foods (e.g., bananas, oats, onions, garlic) may help promote a healthy gut microbiota balance and reduce inflammation in colitis patients.
- **Hydration:** Maintaining adequate hydration by consuming plenty of fluids, such as water, herbal teas, and electrolyte-rich beverages, can help prevent dehydration, support bowel function, and alleviate symptoms of constipation or diarrhea.
- **Small, Frequent Meals:** Eating smaller, more frequent meals throughout the day, rather than large meals, can help prevent abdominal distension, bloating, and discomfort in colitis patients, promoting better digestion and symptom management.

Stress Management

Stress management techniques are essential for reducing stress-related exacerbations of colitis symptoms and promoting overall well-being. Strategies may include:

- **Mindfulness and Relaxation Techniques:** Practicing mindfulness meditation, deep breathing exercises, progressive muscle relaxation, or guided imagery can help reduce stress, promote relaxation, and alleviate symptoms of anxiety or depression.
- **Regular Exercise:** Engaging in regular physical activity, such as walking, jogging, yoga, swimming, or cycling, can help reduce stress, improve mood, enhance

cardiovascular fitness, and promote overall health and well-being in colitis patients.
- **Stress Reduction Strategies:** Identifying stress triggers, practicing time management, setting realistic goals, establishing boundaries, and seeking social support can help individuals cope with stress more effectively and reduce its impact on colitis symptoms.

Smoking Cessation

Smoking has been associated with an increased risk of developing Crohn's disease and may exacerbate symptoms and disease activity in colitis patients. Therefore, smoking cessation is strongly recommended for individuals with colitis to improve disease outcomes and reduce the risk of complications.

Adequate Sleep

Prioritizing adequate sleep and establishing healthy sleep hygiene practices are important for managing colitis symptoms and promoting overall health. Recommendations for improving sleep include:

- **Consistent Sleep Schedule:** Maintaining a consistent sleep schedule by going to bed and waking up at the same time each day can help regulate the body's internal clock and promote restful sleep.
- **Creating a Relaxing Sleep Environment:** Creating a comfortable, quiet, and dark sleep environment, minimizing noise and distractions, and avoiding electronic devices before bedtime can help facilitate relaxation and improve sleep quality.
- **Limiting Stimulants:** Avoiding stimulants such as caffeine, nicotine, and heavy meals close to bedtime can help promote better sleep quality and reduce the risk of nocturnal symptoms in colitis patients.

Medication Adherence

Adhering to prescribed medication regimens is essential for managing colitis symptoms, preventing disease flares, and optimizing treatment outcomes. Patients should:

- **Follow Treatment Plans:** Follow their healthcare provider's recommendations regarding medication dosages, frequencies, and administration routes, and report any concerns or side effects promptly.
- **Attend Regular Follow-Up Visits:** Attend scheduled follow-up appointments with healthcare providers for monitoring disease activity, adjusting treatment regimens as needed, and addressing any questions or concerns about medication adherence or management strategies.

In conclusion, lifestyle modifications are integral to the management of colitis, complementing medical therapies and promoting overall health and well-being. Dietary modifications, stress management techniques, smoking cessation, adequate sleep, and medication adherence are essential components of a comprehensive approach to colitis management, helping individuals optimize symptom control, reduce disease activity, and improve quality of life. Healthcare providers should work collaboratively with patients to develop personalized lifestyle modification plans tailored to their individual needs, preferences, and goals.

Screening and Surveillance

Screening and surveillance strategies are essential components of the management of colitis, including ulcerative colitis (UC),

Crohn's disease, and other inflammatory bowel diseases (IBD). These strategies aim to detect complications, monitor disease activity, and reduce the risk of colorectal cancer (CRC) and other long-term complications associated with colitis. In this section, we explore the principles and recommendations for screening and surveillance in colitis patients.

Principles of Screening and Surveillance

Screening and surveillance in colitis patients are guided by several key principles:

- **Early Detection:** Early detection of complications, such as dysplasia or CRC, allows for timely intervention and improved treatment outcomes.
- **Risk Stratification:** Risk stratification helps identify patients at higher risk for complications, guiding the frequency and intensity of surveillance efforts.
- **Multidisciplinary Approach:** Collaboration among gastroenterologists, colorectal surgeons, pathologists, and other healthcare providers is essential for comprehensive screening and surveillance in colitis patients.
- **Patient Education:** Patient education about the importance of screening and surveillance, as well as adherence to recommended protocols, is crucial for optimizing outcomes.

Screening for Colorectal Cancer

Colorectal cancer (CRC) is a significant long-term complication of colitis, particularly in patients with longstanding and extensive disease involvement. Screening for CRC in colitis patients typically involves:

- **Colonoscopy:** Colonoscopy is the gold standard for CRC screening and surveillance in colitis patients, allowing

direct visualization of the colonic mucosa, detection of dysplastic lesions, and targeted biopsies for histological evaluation.
- **Interval of Surveillance:** The interval between surveillance colonoscopies depends on several factors, including disease duration, extent, severity, and presence of dysplasia. Patients with extensive colitis or a history of dysplasia may require more frequent surveillance.
- **Chromoendoscopy and Advanced Imaging:** Chromoendoscopy, virtual chromoendoscopy (e.g., narrow-band imaging), and other advanced imaging techniques may enhance the detection of dysplastic lesions and improve the accuracy of surveillance colonoscopy in colitis patients.

Surveillance for Dysplasia

Dysplasia is a precursor lesion to CRC in colitis patients, and surveillance efforts aim to detect and manage dysplastic lesions early. Surveillance for dysplasia typically involves:

- **Random Biopsies:** Random biopsies of the colonic mucosa are often performed during surveillance colonoscopy to detect microscopic dysplasia in areas of apparent normal mucosa.
- **Targeted Biopsies:** Targeted biopsies of suspicious lesions, such as nodules, plaques, or areas of mucosal irregularity, are performed to confirm the presence and grade of dysplasia.
- **Histological Evaluation:** Histological evaluation of biopsy specimens by experienced pathologists is essential for accurate diagnosis and grading of dysplasia, guiding treatment decisions and surveillance intervals.

Surveillance for Extraintestinal Manifestations

In addition to CRC surveillance, colitis patients may

require surveillance for extraintestinal manifestations (EIMs) associated with the disease, such as arthritis, dermatologic conditions, ocular manifestations, hepatobiliary disorders, and renal/urologic complications. Surveillance for EIMs involves regular clinical assessments, targeted investigations (e.g., ophthalmologic evaluation, liver function tests), and collaboration with specialists as needed.

Patient Education and Adherence

Patient education about the importance of screening and surveillance, as well as adherence to recommended protocols, is critical for optimizing outcomes in colitis patients. Healthcare providers should provide clear explanations of the rationale for screening and surveillance, discuss potential risks and benefits, address any concerns or misconceptions, and encourage active participation in the screening process.

In conclusion, screening and surveillance are essential components of the management of colitis, facilitating early detection of complications, monitoring disease activity, and reducing the risk of CRC and other long-term complications. Guided by principles such as early detection, risk stratification, multidisciplinary collaboration, and patient education, screening and surveillance efforts aim to optimize outcomes and improve the quality of life for colitis patients. Regular communication, shared decision-making, and ongoing support from healthcare providers are crucial for promoting adherence to screening protocols and ensuring comprehensive care for individuals with colitis.

Early Intervention Strategies

Early intervention strategies are critical components of the management of colitis, including ulcerative colitis (UC),

Crohn's disease, and other inflammatory bowel diseases (IBD). These strategies aim to identify and address disease activity promptly, optimize treatment outcomes, prevent complications, and improve long-term prognosis. In this section, we explore various early intervention strategies employed in the management of colitis.

Prompt Recognition of Symptoms

Prompt recognition of colitis symptoms is essential for early intervention and optimal disease management. Healthcare providers should educate patients about common symptoms of colitis, such as abdominal pain, diarrhea, rectal bleeding, urgency, fatigue, and weight loss, and encourage them to seek medical attention if symptoms worsen or new symptoms develop. Early identification of disease flares allows for timely adjustments to treatment regimens and minimizes the risk of disease progression or complications.

Regular Monitoring and Follow-Up

Regular monitoring and follow-up appointments with healthcare providers are essential for assessing disease activity, monitoring treatment response, and detecting potential complications in colitis patients. Patients should adhere to scheduled appointments and undergo clinical evaluations, laboratory tests, and imaging studies as recommended by their healthcare team. Close monitoring facilitates early intervention, optimization of treatment regimens, and prevention of disease relapses or exacerbations.

Biomarker Monitoring

Biomarker monitoring plays a valuable role in assessing disease activity, predicting treatment response, and guiding therapeutic decisions in colitis patients. Common biomarkers used in colitis management include:

- **C-reactive Protein (CRP) and Erythrocyte Sedimentation Rate (ESR):** Elevated levels of CRP and ESR are indicative of systemic inflammation and may correlate with disease activity in colitis patients. Monitoring these biomarkers can help assess treatment response and guide decisions regarding escalation or modification of therapy.
- **Fecal Calprotectin:** Fecal calprotectin is a sensitive marker of intestinal inflammation and mucosal damage in colitis patients. Regular monitoring of fecal calprotectin levels allows for noninvasive assessment of disease activity and response to treatment, facilitating early intervention and optimization of therapy.
- **Blood Counts:** Complete blood counts, including white blood cell count, hemoglobin, and platelet count, provide valuable information about systemic inflammation, anemia, and thrombocytosis in colitis patients, guiding treatment decisions and monitoring for potential complications.

Treatment Optimization

Early intervention strategies involve optimizing treatment regimens to achieve and maintain disease remission, minimize symptoms, and prevent disease flares or complications. Treatment optimization strategies may include:

- **Pharmacological Therapies:** Adjusting medication dosages, frequencies, or formulations to achieve optimal disease control while minimizing treatment-related side effects.
- **Biologic Therapies:** Initiating or switching to biologic therapies, such as tumor necrosis factor (TNF) alpha inhibitors, vedolizumab, or ustekinumab, in patients with moderate to severe colitis refractory to conventional therapies or at high risk of disease

progression.
- **Immunomodulators:** Adding immunomodulatory agents, such as thiopurines (azathioprine, mercaptopurine) or methotrexate, to induce or maintain remission in colitis patients with inadequate response to conventional therapies or biologic agents.
- **Surgical Consultation:** Considering surgical intervention, such as colectomy or strictureplasty, in colitis patients with complications, refractory disease, or dysplasia not amenable to medical therapy.

Patient Education and Self-Management

Patient education and self-management strategies empower colitis patients to actively participate in their care, recognize signs of disease activity, and adhere to treatment regimens. Healthcare providers should provide comprehensive education about colitis, treatment options, medication adherence, dietary modifications, stress management techniques, and when to seek medical attention for worsening symptoms. Encouraging patients to keep symptom diaries, monitor biomarkers, and engage in healthy lifestyle practices facilitates early intervention and improves long-term outcomes.

In conclusion, early intervention strategies are essential for optimizing the management of colitis, minimizing disease activity, preventing complications, and improving long-term prognosis. Prompt recognition of symptoms, regular monitoring, biomarker assessment, treatment optimization, and patient education are key components of early intervention efforts in colitis management. Multidisciplinary collaboration, shared decision-making, and ongoing support from healthcare providers are essential for implementing early intervention strategies and promoting optimal outcomes in colitis patients.

Management of Comorbidities

Colitis, encompassing conditions like ulcerative colitis (UC), Crohn's disease, and other inflammatory bowel diseases (IBD), often coexists with various comorbidities. Managing these comorbidities is crucial for optimizing overall health, treatment outcomes, and quality of life in colitis patients. Here, we delve into strategies for identifying, assessing, and managing comorbidities in individuals with colitis.

Identification and Assessment

Identifying and assessing comorbidities in colitis patients is a foundational step in their management. This involves:

- **Thorough Medical History:** Obtaining a comprehensive medical history helps uncover past medical conditions, surgeries, medications, family history, lifestyle factors, and psychosocial aspects that may contribute to or be affected by comorbidities.
- **Clinical Evaluation:** Conducting a detailed physical examination, including vital signs assessment, evaluation of gastrointestinal symptoms, extraintestinal manifestations, nutritional status, and signs of complications, aids in identifying potential comorbidities and assessing their severity.
- **Screening Tools and Investigations:** Employing screening tools, questionnaires, laboratory tests, imaging studies, and specialized evaluations (e.g., bone densitometry, ophthalmologic assessments) can facilitate the detection and evaluation of specific comorbidities, such as osteoporosis, arthritis, liver disease, uveitis, or psychological disorders, in colitis patients.

Multidisciplinary Management

A multidisciplinary approach involving gastroenterologists, primary care physicians, specialists (e.g., rheumatologists, dermatologists, ophthalmologists), nurses, dietitians, mental health professionals, and other allied health professionals is essential for comprehensive management of comorbidities in colitis patients. Collaboration among these experts allows for coordinated efforts, knowledge sharing, addressing complex medical issues, and optimizing treatment outcomes through a holistic patient care approach.

Tailored Treatment Approaches

Tailoring treatment approaches to address the unique needs and challenges associated with specific comorbidities is vital. This may involve:

- **Individualized Therapeutic Plans:** Developing individualized treatment plans that consider the presence of comorbidities, potential drug interactions, and the overall health status of the patient.
- **Optimizing Disease Management:** Ensuring optimal management of colitis itself through appropriate medication, lifestyle modifications, and regular monitoring, which can indirectly benefit the management of comorbidities.
- **Coordinated Care:** Coordinating care among different specialties to address the diverse needs of patients with multiple comorbidities, ensuring seamless communication and collaboration in their management.

Lifestyle Modifications

Encouraging and supporting lifestyle modifications can help manage and prevent certain comorbidities in colitis patients. This may include:

- **Healthy Diet:** Promoting a balanced diet rich in nutrients, fiber, and hydration while avoiding trigger foods can support overall health and help manage conditions like obesity, malnutrition, and cardiovascular disease.
- **Regular Exercise:** Encouraging regular physical activity tailored to the patient's abilities and preferences can improve cardiovascular health, muscle strength, flexibility, and mental well-being.
- **Stress Management:** Teaching stress management techniques such as mindfulness, relaxation exercises, and cognitive-behavioral strategies can help mitigate the impact of stress on both colitis and comorbidities like anxiety and depression.

Regular Monitoring and Follow-Up

Regular monitoring and follow-up are essential to assess the progression of comorbidities, evaluate treatment effectiveness, and adjust management strategies as needed. This includes periodic clinical assessments, laboratory tests, imaging studies, and specialist consultations to ensure timely intervention and optimization of care.

In conclusion, the management of comorbidities in colitis patients requires a comprehensive and multidisciplinary approach tailored to individual needs. Identifying comorbidities early, coordinating care among different specialties, optimizing treatment plans, promoting healthy lifestyle modifications, and ensuring regular monitoring are key strategies in effectively managing comorbidities and improving outcomes for colitis patients.

CHAPTER 9: FUTURE DIRECTIONS AND RESEARCH FRONTIERS

Advances in Precision Medicine

Precision medicine, also known as personalized medicine, is a rapidly evolving approach to healthcare that takes into account individual differences in genes, environment, and lifestyle for each person. In the context of colitis and inflammatory bowel diseases (IBD), precision medicine holds great promise for improving diagnosis, treatment, and management strategies. In this section, we will explore the recent advances in precision medicine and their impact on colitis.

Genomic Sequencing and Genetic Markers

Genomic sequencing technologies have revolutionized our ability to understand the genetic basis of diseases, including colitis. Advances in sequencing techniques, such as whole-genome sequencing and genome-wide association studies (GWAS), have enabled the identification of genetic variants associated with colitis susceptibility, disease progression, and treatment response. These genetic markers provide valuable insights into the underlying mechanisms of colitis and offer opportunities for targeted therapies.

Pharmacogenomics

Pharmacogenomics investigates how genetic variations influence an individual's response to drugs. By identifying genetic markers associated with drug metabolism, efficacy, and toxicity, pharmacogenomics allows for the customization of drug therapies to maximize benefits and minimize adverse effects in colitis patients. For example, genetic testing can help predict which patients are more likely to respond to certain medications, such as anti-TNF biologics, and adjust dosages accordingly.

Microbiome Profiling

The gut microbiome plays a crucial role in the pathogenesis of colitis, influencing inflammation, immune responses, and treatment outcomes. Recent advancements in high-throughput sequencing technologies have enabled detailed characterization of the gut microbiome composition in colitis patients. Microbiome profiling allows for the identification of microbial signatures associated with disease severity, treatment response, and disease progression, paving the way for microbiome-based therapies and interventions.

Biomarker Discovery

Precision medicine relies on the identification of biomarkers—measurable indicators of biological processes or disease states—that can inform diagnosis, prognosis, and treatment decisions. In colitis, biomarkers such as fecal calprotectin, C-reactive protein (CRP), and various cytokines have been identified as useful indicators of disease activity, inflammation, and response to therapy. Ongoing research aims to discover novel biomarkers that can improve the accuracy of diagnosis and prediction of disease course in colitis patients.

Artificial Intelligence and Machine Learning

Artificial intelligence (AI) and machine learning algorithms have the potential to transform precision medicine by analyzing vast amounts of multidimensional data, including genomic, clinical, and imaging data. AI-based approaches can identify patterns, correlations, and predictive models that aid in diagnosis, risk stratification, and treatment optimization in colitis. Machine learning algorithms can also facilitate the development of personalized treatment regimens tailored to individual patient characteristics.

Telemedicine and Digital Health Technologies

The integration of telemedicine and digital health technologies enhances the delivery of precision medicine in colitis care. Telemedicine platforms enable remote monitoring, teleconsultations, and patient engagement, facilitating continuous data collection and real-time communication between patients and healthcare providers. Digital health tools, such as smartphone apps and wearable devices, empower patients to track symptoms, monitor medication adherence, and participate in self-management strategies, contributing to personalized and proactive healthcare delivery.

In conclusion, advances in precision medicine have the potential to revolutionize the management of colitis by tailoring treatment strategies to the individual characteristics of each patient. Genomic sequencing, pharmacogenomics, microbiome profiling, biomarker discovery, artificial intelligence, telemedicine, and digital health technologies collectively contribute to a more personalized and effective approach to diagnosing, treating, and managing colitis. As research in precision medicine continues to advance, it holds promise for improving outcomes and quality of life for colitis patients.

Novel Therapeutic Targets

Identifying novel therapeutic targets is essential for advancing the treatment options available for colitis and inflammatory bowel diseases (IBD). Novel therapeutic targets represent specific molecular pathways or cellular mechanisms involved in the pathogenesis of colitis, offering opportunities for the development of innovative and targeted therapies. In this section, we will explore some of the promising novel therapeutic targets for colitis.

Gut Barrier Integrity

Maintaining the integrity of the gut barrier is critical for preventing the entry of harmful substances and pathogens into the intestinal mucosa. Disruption of the gut barrier is associated with increased intestinal permeability and inflammation in colitis. Novel therapeutic targets aimed at enhancing gut barrier function include tight junction proteins, mucin production, and intestinal epithelial cell regeneration pathways.

Innate Immune Activation

The innate immune system plays a crucial role in initiating and regulating the inflammatory response in colitis. Targeting innate immune activation pathways, such as Toll-like receptors (TLRs), NOD-like receptors (NLRs), and inflammasomes, represents a promising approach for modulating inflammation and restoring immune homeostasis in colitis. Small molecule inhibitors and biologic agents targeting these pathways are currently under investigation.

Autophagy Regulation

Autophagy is a cellular process involved in the clearance of damaged organelles and intracellular pathogens, as well as the regulation of inflammation. Dysregulation of autophagy has been implicated in the pathogenesis of colitis. Targeting autophagy regulatory pathways, such as the mTOR signaling pathway and autophagy-related proteins, holds potential for modulating inflammation and promoting intestinal tissue repair in colitis.

Gut Microbiota Modulation

The gut microbiota plays a crucial role in the pathogenesis of colitis, influencing immune responses, inflammation, and epithelial barrier function. Modulating the composition and activity of the gut microbiota through targeted interventions, such as probiotics, prebiotics, and fecal microbiota transplantation (FMT), represents a promising therapeutic approach for colitis. Identifying specific microbial species or metabolites associated with disease pathogenesis may lead to the development of microbiome-targeted therapies.

Neuroimmune Interactions

The bidirectional communication between the nervous system and the immune system, known as the neuroimmune axis, plays a significant role in regulating intestinal inflammation and mucosal immunity. Targeting neuroimmune interactions, such as the vagus nerve and neurotransmitter pathways, may offer novel therapeutic opportunities for modulating inflammation and restoring immune balance in colitis.

Epigenetic Modifications

Epigenetic modifications, such as DNA methylation, histone modifications, and non-coding RNA regulation, play a critical role in regulating gene expression and cellular function in colitis. Targeting epigenetic mechanisms involved in the dysregulation of inflammatory pathways may offer novel therapeutic strategies for colitis. Epigenetic modifiers and histone deacetylase inhibitors are currently being investigated as potential therapeutic agents.

In conclusion, identifying and targeting novel therapeutic targets is essential for advancing the treatment of colitis. Novel therapeutic targets, including gut barrier integrity, innate immune activation, autophagy regulation, gut microbiota modulation, neuroimmune interactions, and epigenetic modifications, offer promising opportunities for developing innovative and targeted therapies for colitis. Further research and clinical trials are needed to validate these targets and translate them into effective treatments for patients with colitis.

Biomarkers for Predicting Disease Course

Biomarkers are measurable indicators of biological processes or disease states that can provide valuable information for predicting the course and outcome of diseases. In the context of colitis and inflammatory bowel diseases (IBD), identifying biomarkers for predicting disease course is essential for guiding treatment decisions, monitoring disease activity, and improving patient outcomes. In this section, we will explore some of the biomarkers that hold promise for predicting the disease course in colitis.

Fecal Calprotectin

Fecal calprotectin is a sensitive biomarker of intestinal inflammation and mucosal damage in colitis. Elevated levels of fecal calprotectin are indicative of active inflammation in the gastrointestinal tract and correlate with disease severity. Monitoring fecal calprotectin levels over time can help predict disease relapse, response to treatment, and the risk of disease complications in colitis patients.

C-Reactive Protein (CRP)

C-reactive protein (CRP) is an acute-phase reactant produced by the liver in response to inflammation. Elevated levels of CRP in the blood are associated with systemic inflammation and disease activity in colitis. Measuring CRP levels can help assess disease severity, monitor response to treatment, and predict the risk of disease complications, such as strictures and fistulas, in colitis patients.

Cytokine Profiles

Cytokines are key mediators of inflammation and immune responses in colitis. Profiling cytokine levels in the blood or mucosal tissues can provide insights into the underlying inflammatory pathways driving disease progression. Elevated levels of pro-inflammatory cytokines, such as tumor necrosis factor-alpha (TNF-alpha), interleukin-6 (IL-6), and interleukin-17 (IL-17), are associated with more severe disease and poorer treatment outcomes in colitis patients.

Genetic Markers

Genetic markers associated with colitis susceptibility and disease progression can help predict the likelihood of developing complications and the response to specific treatments. Common genetic variants, such as those in the NOD2 and IL23R genes, have been linked to an increased risk of colitis and can serve as prognostic biomarkers for disease course and treatment response.

Endoscopic and Histologic Findings

Endoscopic evaluation and histologic examination of intestinal tissue provide valuable information about disease activity, severity, and mucosal healing in colitis. Biomarkers such as mucosal ulceration, crypt abscesses, and architectural changes observed during endoscopy and histology can help predict disease relapse, response to therapy, and long-term outcomes in colitis patients.

Microbial Biomarkers

The composition and diversity of the gut microbiota are altered in colitis, and specific microbial signatures may be associated with disease activity and progression. Identifying microbial biomarkers, such as changes in microbial composition or metabolite profiles, can help predict disease flares, treatment response, and the risk of disease complications in colitis patients.

In conclusion, identifying biomarkers for predicting the disease course is crucial for optimizing the management of colitis and improving patient outcomes. Fecal calprotectin, CRP, cytokine profiles, genetic markers, endoscopic and histologic findings, and microbial biomarkers offer valuable insights into disease activity, severity, and treatment response in colitis patients. Integrating these biomarkers into clinical practice can help personalize treatment strategies, monitor disease progression, and improve the overall care of patients with colitis. Continued research and validation of biomarkers are needed to further enhance their utility in predicting the disease course in colitis.

CHAPTER 10: HOLISTIC HEALTH AND COLITIS MANAGEMENT

Mind-Body Connection

The mind-body connection refers to the intricate relationship between mental and physical health, where the state of one's mind influences the state of their body, and vice versa. In the context of colitis and inflammatory bowel diseases (IBD), understanding and harnessing the mind-body connection can play a significant role in managing symptoms and improving overall well-being. In this section, we will explore the importance of the mind-body connection in colitis and strategies for promoting holistic health.

Stress and Its Impact on Colitis

Chronic stress can exacerbate symptoms and trigger flare-ups in colitis patients. Stress activates the body's "fight or flight" response, leading to increased inflammation and immune activation in the gastrointestinal tract. Moreover, stress can disrupt gut motility and barrier function, further worsening symptoms of colitis. Recognizing stress triggers and implementing stress-reduction techniques, such as mindfulness meditation and relaxation exercises, can help mitigate the impact of stress on colitis symptoms.

Psychological Factors and Disease Management

Psychological factors, including anxiety, depression, and negative coping mechanisms, can significantly impact disease management and treatment outcomes in colitis patients. Psychological distress can exacerbate symptoms, reduce medication adherence, and impair quality of life. Incorporating psychological interventions, such as cognitive-behavioral therapy (CBT) and stress management techniques, into the treatment plan can improve psychological well-being and enhance coping skills in colitis patients.

Gut-Brain Axis and Neurotransmitter Regulation

The gut-brain axis represents bidirectional communication between the gut and the central nervous system, involving hormonal, neural, and immune pathways. Neurotransmitters, such as serotonin and gamma-aminobutyric acid (GABA), produced in the gut play a crucial role in regulating mood, cognition, and gastrointestinal function. Imbalances in neurotransmitter levels can contribute to both gastrointestinal symptoms and psychological disorders in colitis patients. Targeting the gut-brain axis through lifestyle modifications, dietary interventions, and gut-directed therapies can promote symbiotic interactions between the gut and the brain, improving both mental and physical health outcomes.

Lifestyle Modifications for Holistic Health

Adopting healthy lifestyle habits, including regular exercise, balanced nutrition, adequate sleep, and stress management, is essential for promoting holistic health in colitis patients.

Physical activity can reduce inflammation, improve gut motility, and enhance mood and cognitive function. A well-balanced diet rich in fiber, fruits, vegetables, and omega-3 fatty acids can support gut health and reduce the risk of disease flares. Prioritizing self-care activities, such as relaxation techniques, hobbies, and social connections, can also contribute to overall well-being and resilience in colitis patients.

Integrative Approaches to Colitis Management

Integrative approaches that combine conventional medical treatments with complementary therapies, such as acupuncture, yoga, and herbal supplements, can address the mind-body connection in colitis management. These modalities aim to promote relaxation, reduce stress, and enhance overall health and quality of life. Integrative care plans tailored to individual patient needs can empower colitis patients to take an active role in their health and well-being, fostering a holistic approach to disease management.

In conclusion, recognizing and nurturing the mind-body connection is essential for optimizing health outcomes in colitis patients. By addressing psychological factors, promoting stress management techniques, and adopting holistic lifestyle modifications, healthcare providers can support colitis patients in achieving greater resilience, symptom control, and overall well-being. Embracing the mind-body connection offers a comprehensive approach to colitis management that honors the interconnectedness of mental and physical health.

Stress Management Techniques

Managing stress is crucial for individuals with colitis as it can help reduce symptom flare-ups, improve overall well-being, and enhance the effectiveness of treatment. In this section, we will explore various stress management techniques that can be beneficial for individuals living with colitis.

Mindfulness Meditation

Mindfulness meditation involves focusing your attention on the present moment without judgment. This practice can help reduce stress and anxiety by promoting relaxation and increasing self-awareness. Colitis patients can benefit from incorporating mindfulness meditation into their daily routine, even if it's just a few minutes of mindful breathing or body scanning.

Deep Breathing Exercises

Deep breathing exercises, such as diaphragmatic breathing or belly breathing, can activate the body's relaxation response, counteracting the physiological effects of stress. Colitis patients can practice deep breathing techniques whenever they feel stressed or anxious, focusing on slow, deep breaths to calm the mind and body.

Progressive Muscle Relaxation (PMR)

Progressive muscle relaxation involves tensing and relaxing different muscle groups in the body to release physical tension and promote relaxation. Colitis patients can practice PMR by systematically tensing and relaxing each muscle group, starting from the toes and working their way up to the head, while focusing on deep breathing and sensations of relaxation.

Yoga and Tai Chi

Yoga and tai chi are mind-body practices that combine physical postures, breath control, and meditation to promote relaxation and reduce stress. Colitis patients can benefit from gentle yoga or tai chi routines designed to improve flexibility, strength, and mental clarity while fostering a sense of calm and balance.

Guided Imagery and Visualization

Guided imagery and visualization involve using mental imagery to evoke feelings of relaxation and well-being. Colitis patients can listen to guided imagery recordings or create their own visualizations, imagining themselves in a peaceful, serene environment or visualizing their body's healing process to promote relaxation and reduce stress.

Journaling and Expressive Writing

Journaling and expressive writing can be therapeutic tools for processing emotions, reducing stress, and gaining insights into one's thoughts and feelings. Colitis patients can use journaling to explore their experiences with the disease, identify stress triggers, and cultivate a sense of gratitude and resilience.

Social Support and Connection

Maintaining social connections and seeking support from friends, family, or support groups can help buffer the effects of stress and provide emotional validation and encouragement. Colitis patients can benefit from sharing their experiences with others who understand their challenges and offering support to fellow patients facing similar struggles.

Time Management and Prioritization

Effective time management and prioritization can help reduce stress by providing structure and organization to daily activities. Colitis patients can benefit from creating realistic schedules, setting achievable goals, and delegating tasks when necessary to avoid feeling overwhelmed and maintain a sense of control.

In conclusion, incorporating stress management techniques into daily life can help colitis patients better cope with the challenges of living with a chronic illness. By practicing mindfulness, deep breathing, progressive muscle relaxation, engaging in mind-body practices like yoga and tai chi, utilizing guided imagery and visualization, journaling, seeking social support, and effectively managing time and priorities, individuals with colitis can reduce stress levels, improve symptom management, and enhance overall quality of life.

Importance of Sleep and Circadian Rhythms

Sleep plays a vital role in maintaining overall health and well-being, including the management of colitis and inflammatory bowel diseases (IBD). In this section, we will explore the importance of sleep and circadian rhythms in relation to colitis and strategies for promoting healthy sleep habits.

Regulation of Circadian Rhythms

Circadian rhythms are 24-hour biological cycles that regulate various physiological processes, including sleep-wake cycles, hormone secretion, metabolism, and immune function. Disruptions to circadian rhythms, such as irregular sleep patterns or shift work, can negatively impact health and increase the risk of chronic diseases, including colitis.

Sleep and Immune Function

Sleep plays a critical role in regulating immune function and inflammation. During sleep, the body undergoes repair and regeneration processes, and the immune system becomes more active in fighting off infections and inflammation. Chronic sleep deprivation or poor sleep quality can impair immune function and exacerbate inflammation in colitis patients.

Impact of Sleep Disturbances on Colitis

Sleep disturbances, such as insomnia, sleep fragmentation, and sleep apnea, are common among individuals with colitis and IBD. These sleep disturbances can worsen disease symptoms, increase inflammation, and contribute to disease flares and relapses. Addressing sleep problems is essential for optimizing disease management and improving quality of life in colitis patients.

Gut-Brain Axis and Sleep

The gut-brain axis plays a crucial role in regulating sleep-wake cycles and circadian rhythms. Bidirectional communication between the gut and the brain influences sleep patterns, mood, and cognitive function. Disruptions to the gut microbiota, intestinal inflammation, and stress can affect sleep quality and contribute to sleep disturbances in colitis patients.

Strategies for Promoting Healthy Sleep Habits

Promoting healthy sleep habits is essential for individuals with colitis to improve sleep quality and overall well-being. Some strategies for promoting healthy sleep habits include:

- Establishing a consistent sleep schedule: Going to bed and waking up at the same time every day helps regulate circadian rhythms and promote better sleep quality.
- Creating a relaxing bedtime routine: Engaging in calming activities before bedtime, such as reading, taking a warm bath, or practicing relaxation techniques, can help signal to the body that it's time to wind down and prepare for sleep.
- Creating a sleep-friendly environment: Creating a comfortable and conducive sleep environment, with a cool, dark, and quiet bedroom, can help facilitate restful sleep.
- Limiting caffeine and alcohol intake: Consuming caffeine and alcohol close to bedtime can disrupt sleep patterns

and lead to poor sleep quality. Limiting intake of these substances in the hours leading up to bedtime can promote better sleep.
- Managing stress and anxiety: Stress and anxiety can interfere with sleep quality. Engaging in stress-reduction techniques, such as mindfulness meditation, deep breathing exercises, or journaling, can help promote relaxation and improve sleep quality.

In conclusion, prioritizing healthy sleep habits and maintaining regular circadian rhythms are essential for managing colitis and promoting overall health and well-being. By understanding the importance of sleep and implementing strategies to improve sleep quality, individuals with colitis can enhance their disease management and quality of life. Working with healthcare providers to address sleep disturbances and prioritize sleep hygiene can lead to better outcomes for colitis patients.

Exercise and Physical Activity Recommendations

Regular exercise and physical activity play a crucial role in managing colitis and promoting overall health and well-being. In this section, we will explore the benefits of exercise for colitis patients and provide recommendations for incorporating physical activity into daily life.

Benefits of Exercise for Colitis

Regular exercise offers numerous benefits for individuals with colitis, including:

- **Reduced Inflammation:** Exercise has anti-inflammatory effects that can help reduce inflammation in the gastrointestinal tract, potentially leading to fewer

disease flares and milder symptoms.
- **Improved Immune Function:** Exercise can enhance immune function, making the body more resilient to infections and reducing the risk of complications in colitis patients.
- **Enhanced Gut Motility:** Physical activity promotes healthy gut motility, reducing the risk of constipation and improving digestive function in colitis patients.
- **Stress Reduction:** Exercise is a natural stress reliever, helping to reduce anxiety, depression, and psychological distress commonly experienced by colitis patients.
- **Weight Management:** Regular exercise can help maintain a healthy weight, which is important for managing colitis symptoms and reducing the risk of disease complications.

Exercise Recommendations for Colitis Patients

Colitis patients should aim to incorporate both aerobic exercise and strength training into their routine. Here are some exercise recommendations for colitis patients:

- **Aerobic Exercise:** Aim for at least 150 minutes of moderate-intensity aerobic exercise or 75 minutes of vigorous-intensity aerobic exercise each week. Activities such as brisk walking, cycling, swimming, or jogging can help improve cardiovascular health and overall fitness.
- **Strength Training:** Include strength training exercises at least two days per week, targeting major muscle groups such as the arms, legs, abdomen, and back. Strength training can help improve muscle strength, endurance, and bone density, reducing the risk of osteoporosis and frailty.
- **Flexibility and Balance Exercises:** Incorporate flexibility and balance exercises, such as yoga, tai chi, or stretching routines, to improve range of motion, posture, and

stability. These exercises can help prevent injuries and improve overall mobility and quality of life.
- **Listen to Your Body:** Be mindful of your body's limitations and listen to any warning signs or symptoms during exercise. If you experience pain, fatigue, or discomfort, modify or stop the activity and consult with your healthcare provider.

Tips for Exercising with Colitis

- **Stay Hydrated:** Drink plenty of water before, during, and after exercise to stay hydrated and prevent dehydration, especially if you experience diarrhea or increased fluid loss due to colitis symptoms.
- **Choose Low-Impact Activities:** If you experience joint pain or discomfort, consider low-impact exercises such as swimming, cycling, or using an elliptical machine to reduce stress on your joints.
- **Plan Ahead:** Schedule exercise sessions at times when you typically feel your best and have the most energy. Listen to your body and adjust your exercise routine as needed based on your symptoms and energy levels.
- **Work with a Healthcare Provider:** Consult with your healthcare provider before starting a new exercise program, especially if you have any underlying health conditions or concerns. They can provide personalized recommendations and guidance based on your individual needs and medical history.

In conclusion, regular exercise and physical activity are essential components of a healthy lifestyle for individuals with colitis. By incorporating aerobic exercise, strength training, flexibility, and balance exercises into their routine, colitis patients can improve their physical fitness, reduce inflammation, manage stress, and enhance overall well-being. Working closely with healthcare providers and listening to their bodies' needs can help colitis patients safely and effectively incorporate exercise into their daily lives.

Dietary Guidelines for Colitis Patients

Diet plays a significant role in managing colitis and inflammatory bowel diseases (IBD), influencing disease symptoms, inflammation levels, and overall gut health. In this section, we will explore dietary guidelines and recommendations for colitis patients to help manage symptoms, promote gut healing, and improve quality of life.

Individualized Approach

Dietary recommendations for colitis patients should be tailored to individual needs, preferences, and tolerances. What works for one person may not work for another, so it's essential to work with a healthcare provider or registered dietitian to develop a personalized nutrition plan based on your specific dietary triggers, symptoms, and nutritional requirements.

Maintain Adequate Nutrition

Colitis patients should strive to maintain adequate nutrition to support overall health and well-being. Focus on consuming a balanced diet that includes a variety of nutrient-rich foods, such as fruits, vegetables, whole grains, lean proteins, and healthy fats. Consider working with a dietitian to ensure you're meeting your nutritional needs, especially if you have dietary restrictions or concerns about certain food groups.

Identify Trigger Foods

Identifying trigger foods that exacerbate colitis symptoms is essential for managing the condition. Keep a food diary to track your diet and symptoms, paying attention to any patterns or correlations between specific foods and flare-ups. Common trigger foods for colitis patients may include spicy foods, high-fiber foods, dairy products, caffeine, alcohol, and processed foods. Once trigger foods are identified, consider eliminating or reducing them from your diet to see if symptoms improve.

Emphasize Gut-Friendly Foods

Incorporating gut-friendly foods into your diet can help promote gut healing and reduce inflammation in colitis patients. Focus on consuming foods that are easy to digest, low in fiber, and gentle on the gastrointestinal tract, such as cooked fruits and vegetables, lean proteins, refined grains, and lactose-free dairy products. Additionally, include foods rich in anti-inflammatory nutrients, such as omega-3 fatty acids, antioxidants, and probiotics, to help support gut health.

Practice Portion Control

Maintaining appropriate portion sizes can help prevent overeating and minimize digestive discomfort in colitis patients. Eat smaller, more frequent meals throughout the day rather than large, heavy meals that may overwhelm the digestive system. Pay attention to portion sizes and listen to your body's hunger and fullness cues to avoid overeating.

Stay Hydrated

Proper hydration is essential for supporting digestion, preventing dehydration, and maintaining overall health in colitis patients. Drink plenty of fluids throughout the day, including water, herbal teas, and electrolyte-rich beverages, to stay hydrated and support optimal hydration levels. Limiting or avoiding caffeinated and carbonated beverages, which can irritate the gastrointestinal tract, may also be beneficial.

Consider Supplements

In some cases, colitis patients may require dietary supplements to address nutrient deficiencies or support gut health. Talk to your healthcare provider or dietitian about potential supplementation options, such as vitamin D, calcium, iron, B vitamins, omega-3 fatty acids, and probiotics, to ensure you're meeting your nutritional needs.

Monitor Symptoms and Adjust Diet Accordingly

Continuously monitor your symptoms and how they respond to dietary changes, making adjustments as needed to optimize symptom management and gut health. Be patient and willing to experiment with different foods and dietary approaches to find what works best for you. Keep communication lines open with your healthcare team to discuss any concerns or questions about your diet and its impact on your colitis symptoms.

In conclusion, following dietary guidelines and recommendations tailored to individual needs is essential for managing colitis effectively. By maintaining adequate nutrition, identifying trigger foods, emphasizing gut-friendly foods, practicing portion control, staying hydrated, considering supplementation, and monitoring symptoms, colitis patients can optimize their diet to support gut healing, reduce inflammation, and improve overall quality of life. Working closely with healthcare providers and registered dietitians can provide valuable guidance and support in developing a personalized nutrition plan that meets individual needs and preferences.

Made in United States
North Haven, CT
08 April 2024